STUDY GUIDE

Pharmacology for the Surgical Technologist

SECOND EDITION

Katherine C. Snyder, CST, BS
Surgical Technology Program Director
Laramie County Community College
Cheyenne, Wyoming

Chris Keegan, CST, MS
Professor and Chair
Surgical Technology and Surgical First Assisting Programs
Vincennes University
Vincennes, Indiana

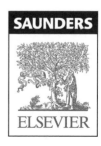

SAUNDERS

ELSEVIER

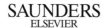

SAUNDERS
ELSEVIER

11830 Westline Industrial Drive
St. Louis, Missouri 63146

STUDY GUIDE FOR PHARMACOLOGY FOR THE SURGICAL   ISBN-13: 978-1-4160-2459-0
TECHNOLOGIST, SECOND EDITION   ISBN-10: 1-4160-2459-X
Copyright © 2006 by Elsevier Inc.

Notice

Knowledge and best practice in this field are constantly changing. As new research and experience broaden our knowledge, changes in practice, treatment, and drug therapy may become necessary or appropriate. Readers are advised to check the most current information provided (i) on procedures featured or (ii) by the manufacturer of each product to be administered, to verify the recommended dose or formula, the method and duration of administration, and contraindications. It is the responsibility of the practitioner, relying on his or her own experience and knowledge of the patient, to make diagnoses, to determine dosages and the best treatment for each individual patient, and to take all appropriate safety precautions. To the fullest extent of the law, neither the Publisher nor the Authors assume any liability for any injury and/or damage to persons or property arising out or related to any use of the material contained in this book.

The Publisher

ISBN-13: 978-1-4160-2459-0
ISBN-10: 1-4160-2459-X

Publisher: Michael Ledbetter
Associate Developmental Editor: Katherine Judge
Publishing Services Manager: Julie Eddy
Project Manager: Kelly E.M. Steinmann
Designer: Julia Dummitt

Printed in the United States of America

Last digit is the print number: 9 8 7 6 5

Contents

Introduction

Welcome to the Study Guide for the second edition of *Pharmacology for the Surgical Technologist*. This Study Guide has been developed to assist students in mastering the vital content covered in the textbook. The effective use of this guide will help you gain a deeper and broader understanding of the material presented. Due to the critical safety issues regarding pharmacology in surgery, it is vital that you learn this information for the long term of your clinical practice rather than for the short term of the next examination in school. Remember that although your short-term goal is to pass the course, your long-term goal is to provide safe surgical patient care. The scrubbed surgical technologist is the last line of defense against medication errors on the sterile field. Thus, it is important that you understand what and how medications are used. This Study Guide is intended to assist you in the process of building a solid foundation of surgical pharmacology knowledge for life so that during your career new information may be added to that foundation.

How to Use the Study Guide

Each chapter is broken down in sections to help you understand and learn the material included. The objectives lay out the information you will learn, and the outline defines the chapter's content. The next section contains exercises and assignments on chapter materials. These exercises require you to use your text and other sources. Here are some tips to enhance your learning:

- When defining the key terms, use complete sentences for your definitions and be precise.
- Reread the chapter to answer the questions.
- In Chapter 3 there are additional math exercises to improve your skills—review examples given in the chapter for each section, which is highlighted for you.
- Critical thinking skills may involve observation and questions at your clinical site.
- Use the CD included with your textbook to answer some of the questions under Utilizing Pharmacology Resources.
- When searching the Internet, use search engines such as Google, Ask Jeeves, and Web Ferret.
- Drug cards are included for you to do additional research on some medications. Use *Mosby's Drug Consult*, the *Physician's Desk Reference*, the Internet, and other sources to complete them.

At the end of many chapters there is a special section titled Advanced Practices. This provides additional material for the surgical technologist who is experienced in the field and acts as the surgical first assistant during procedures. However, it may be of interest to you as an entry-level surgical technology student as well. This information may provide additional classroom discussion, extra credit, and the opportunity for critical thinking. Questions and references for the Advanced Practices sections are found after the chapter quiz.

1 Basic Pharmacology

CHAPTER OBJECTIVES

After completing this chapter, you should be able to:
1. Define terms and abbreviations related to pharmacology.
2. List sources of drugs and give an example of each.
3. List four drug classification categories and identify several subcategories in each.
4. Discuss medication orders used in surgery.
5. List the parts of a medication order.
6. Describe the drug distribution systems used in hospitals.
7. List types of drug forms.
8. Discuss the medication administration routes used in surgery.
9. Describe the four processes of pharmacokinetics.
10. Discuss aspects of pharmacodynamics.

CHAPTER OUTLINE

  I. Drug Sources
     A. Natural
        1. Plants
        2. Animals
        3. Minerals
     B. Chemical Synthesis
        1. Synthetic
        2. Semisynthetic
     C. Biotechnology
 II. Drug Classifications
III. Medication Orders
     A. Prescriptions
     B. Hospital Medication Orders
 IV. Drug Distribution Systems
  V. Drug Forms or Preparations
     A. Solids
     B. Semisolids
     C. Liquids
     D. Gases
 VI. Drug Administration Routes
VII. Pharmacokinetics
     A. Absorption
     B. Distribution
     C. Metabolism
     D. Excretion
VIII. Pharmacodynamics
  IX. Advanced Practices for the Surgical First Assistant

CHAPTER CONTENT MASTERY

Learning the Language (Key Terms)
Using your textbook or a standard medical dictionary, look up and write the definition of each term.

1. Absorption: _____

2. Adverse effect: _____

1

3. Agonist: _____

4. Antagonist: _____

5. Bioavailability: _____

6. Biotechnology: _____

7. Biotransformation: _____

8. Bolus: _____

9. Contraindication: _____

10. Distribution: _____

11. Duration: _____

12. Emulsion: _____

13. Enteral: _____

14. Excretion: _____

15. Hypersensitivity: _____

16. Idiosyncratic effect: _____

17. Indication: _____

18. Local effect: _____

19. Metabolism: _____

20. Onset: _____

21. Parenteral: _____

22. Pharmacodynamics: _____

23. Pharmacokinetics: _____

24. Plasma protein binding: _____

25. Reconstituted: _____

26. Side effects: _____

27. Solubility: _____

28. Solution: _____

29. Suspension: _____

30. Synergist: _____

31. Systemic effect: _____

32. Topical: _____

Chapter Review Questions

1. What are the three major sources of drugs used today?

    a. _____

    b. _____

    c. _____

2. State an example of a medication from each major source.

    a. _____

    b. _____

    c. _____

3. How are drug classification categories helpful? _____

    _____

4. What types of drug orders are used in surgery? _____

    _____

5. If you are currently in your clinical rotation or if you have made a field trip to a local hospital, describe

    the drug distribution system used in that clinical facility. _____

    _____

6. If you are currently in your clinical rotation, which drug forms/preparations and administration routes

    have you seen used in surgery? _____

    _____

7. How does the body process drugs? _____

    _____

8. What is a side effect? An adverse effect? An idiosyncratic effect? Give an example of each.

    _____

    _____

    _____

Critical Thinking

Scenario 1

Mrs. Lopez is a 52-year-old woman with type 1 diabetes. She has been taking insulin for 10 years. Recently, she has developed some reactivity to the insulin she has always taken. Her physician has prescribed Humulin instead of regular insulin. Humulin is a drug that has been developed using biotechnology.

1. What might she have been reacting to in the regular insulin? _____

    _____

2. Why might switching to Humulin solve her problem? _____

    _____

3. How is Humulin produced using biotechnology? _____

    _____

Chapter **1** **Basic Pharmacology**

Scenario 2

Mr. Dhang is a 75-year-old man taking Coumadin for recurrent deep vein thrombosis (DVT). He recently began experiencing frequent, almost daily, headaches but has not consulted his physician. He has started taking aspirin to treat his headaches.

1. Why is taking aspirin while on Coumadin a problem? _____

    _____

2. How does the presence of aspirin alter the effect of Coumadin? _____

    _____

3. Which adverse effects might you expect to see? _____

    _____

Utilizing Pharmacology Resources

1. Select one pharmacology resource and complete a medication information worksheet for human insulin (Humulin).
2. Select a second pharmacology resource and complete a medication information worksheet for meperidine (Demerol).
3. Write an essay comparing the advantages and disadvantages of the two resources you selected.
4. Call a local hospital pharmacy and request an interview with a staff pharmacist. Ask the pharmacist to describe his or her role as a pharmacology resource for you as a graduate surgical technologist working in surgery. Write an essay describing how you might use a pharmacist as a resource person during clinical practice.

Internet Exercises

1. Using your favorite search engine, look up any medication listed in the textbook.

    a. How many "hits" did you get? _____
    b. List five of the websites the search engine found for you.

    _____

    _____

    _____

    _____

    _____

    c. Which of the listed websites do you think would be the most reliable?

    _____

    d. Visit three of the websites you think are most reliable.
    e. Which of the sites you visited provided the most helpful information?

    _____

2. Complete a medication information worksheet based on the information you found from that website. (Keep in mind the website may not contain all the information listed on the worksheet.)

1. Define the term *biotechnology*. _____

   _____

2. List one of the three major sources of medications. _____
3. Which of the following is NOT one of the four major drug classification categories?
   A. Affected body system
   B. Chemical type
   C. Narcotic antagonist
   D. Therapeutic action

4. Discuss a PRN drug order as used in surgery. _____

   _____

5. List one part of a medication order. _____

   _____

6. Describe one type of drug distribution system used in a hospital. _____

   _____

7. Which of the following is NOT one of the four drug forms?
   A. Cream
   B. Gas
   C. Liquid
   D. Solid

8. Discuss the parenteral administration route used in surgery. _____

   _____

9. List one of the four processes of pharmacokinetics. _____

   _____

10. Define the term *side effect*. _____

   _____

ADVANCED PRACTICES CONTENT MASTERY

Learning the Language (Key Terms)

Using your textbook or a standard medical dictionary, look up and write the definition of each term.
1. Tolerance:

   _____

2. Therapeutic levels:

   _____

3. Tachyphylaxis:

   _____

4. Drug dependence:

   _____

Advanced Practices Chapter Review Questions

1. When writing a medication order, it is the surgical assistant's duty to
   A. Sign and initial the order for the physician
   B. Have the physician verify, clarify, and sign it
   C. Verify the four components are present on the order
   D. Have the physician sign it before checking the order
2. Prescription pads are
   A. Signed in advance by the physician
   B. Kept in an area where they can be easily accessed
   C. Signed and initialed by the surgical assistant
   D. Kept in a secure place
3. Which of the following has been added to the four basic vital signs?
   A. Pain
   B. Heart rate
   C. Respirations
   D. Pupil reaction
4. A type of tolerance that develops quickly and can occur following one or two doses is
   A. Tachyphylaxis
   B. Catalysis
   C. Autotoxemia
   D. Anaphylaxis

CHAPTER REFERENCES

Hopper T: Mosby's Pharmacy Technician Principles and Practice. St Louis, WB Saunders, 2004.
Mosby's Drug Consult. St Louis, Elsevier, 2005.
Physician's Desk Reference, 59th ed. Montvale, NJ, Medical Economics, Inc, 2005.
Saeb-Parsy K, Assomull RG, Khan FZ, et al: Instant Pharmacology. Chichester, England, Wiley and Sons, 1999.
www.bumc.bu.edu/Dept/Content.aspx?DepartmentID=65&PageID=7797
www.channel1.com/users/medlan/pharm/pharm.htm
www.dea.gov
www.jcaho.org
www.nurse-prescriber.co.uk/education/modules/pharmacology/pharmacy3.htm
www.pharmacology-info.com/
www.physpharm.fmd.uwo.ca/www/resource.html
www.pyxis.com/

ADVANCED PRACTICES CHAPTER REFERENCES

Gutierrez K: Pharmacotherapeutics: Clinical Decision-Making in Nursing. Philadelphia, WB Saunders, 1999.
Kee JL, Hayes ER: Pharmacology: A Nursing Process Approach, 3rd ed. Philadelphia, WB Saunders, 2000.

Medication Development, Regulation, and Resources

CHAPTER OBJECTIVES

After completing this chapter, you should be able to:
1. Discuss federal and state roles in regulating drugs.
2. Define medication development and testing.
3. Discuss pharmacogenetics and pharmacogenomics.
4. Distinguish brand, generic, and chemical medication names.
5. List information found on medication labels.
6. Obtain medication information from pharmacology resources.

CHAPTER OUTLINE

I. Medication Regulation
   A. Federal Laws
      1. Pure Food and Drug Act
      2. Food, Drug, and Cosmetic Act
      3. Durham-Humphrey Amendments
         a. Prescription Medications
         b. Over-The-Counter (OTC) Medications
      4. Controlled Substances Act
      5. Drug Enforcement Administration (DEA)
   B. Federal Agencies
      1. Occupational Safety and Health Administration (OSHA)
      2. Centers for Disease Control and Prevention (CDC)
   C. State Practice Acts
   D. Local Policies
   E. Joint Commission on Accreditation of Healthcare Organizations (JCAHO)
II. Drug Development
   A. Testing
      1. FDA Regulation
      2. FDA Pregnancy Categories
      3. Pharmacogenetic
   B. Marketing
   C. Medication Labeling
      1. Verifying Medication
      2. Label Information
III. Medication References
   A. Physician's Desk Reference (PDR)
   B. United States Pharmacopoeia and National Formulary (USP/NF)
   C. American Hospital Formulary Service (AHFS) Drug Information
   D. The Medical Letter
   E. Drug Facts and Comparisons
   F. Hospital Pharmacist
   G. Databases

CHAPTER CONTENT MASTERY

Learning the Language (Key Terms)

Using your textbook or a standard medical dictionary, look up and write the definition of each term.

1. AHFS drug information: _____

2. Contraindication: _____

7

3. Controlled substances: _____

4. DEA: _____

5. *Drug Facts and Comparisons:* _____

6. FDA: _____

7. Indication: _____

8. JCAHO: _____

9. Narcotics: _____

10. OTC: _____

11. *PDR:* _____

12. Pharmacogenetics/pharmacogenomics: _____

_____

13. Prescription drugs: _____

14. *USP/NF:* _____

Chapter Review Questions

1. How does the federal government regulate medications?

   _____

2. What is the significance of the Pure Food and Drug Act of 1906?

   _____

3. What is the role of the FDA in drug regulation?

   _____

4. Why is the separation of drugs into five schedules important?

   _____

5. What is the role of JCAHO in medication regulation? OSHA? CDC?

   _____

   _____

   _____

6. Use at least two different clinical medication references to look up indications for and side effects of the following medications:

   a. Heparin sodium _____

   _____

   b. Lasix _____

   _____

   c. Keflin _____

   _____

7. Why is it important for the surgical technologist to have an understanding of medications, as he or she does not directly administer them to the patient?

   _____

   _____

Critical Thinking

1. How does the DEA affect clinical practice?

   _____

   _____

2. Name three medications that the surgeon uses during a procedure that are prepared on the back table.

   _____

   _____

3. How are medications for procedures obtained at your clinical site?

   _____

Chapter **2** Medication Development, Regulation, and Resources

Scenario

The surgery is scheduled as an excision of a cyst from the right lower back. The surgeon requests Xylocaine 1% with epinephrine, Demerol, and Versed for this local procedure.

1. What are the generic names for these medications? _____

   _____

2. Xylocaine is available in what strengths (in addition to the 1%)? _____

   _____

3. Which of these medications are narcotics? What are their controlled substance schedules?

   _____

   _____

   _____

4. Which of the medications would have a red label? Why? _____

   _____

Visual Exercises

Medication Label Identification

Look at the two heparin sodium labels pictured and answer the following questions.

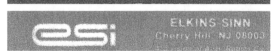 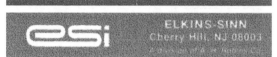

From Kee JL, Marshall SM: Clinical Calculations: With Applications to General and Specialty Areas, 5th ed. St Louis, Saunders, 2000.

1. From what source is the heparin sodium derived? _____
2. What are the strengths of the medications? Are they the same? How do you know?

   _____

   _____

3. By what route is this medication administered to the patient? _____

_____

4. How much of the medication is in each container?

_____

Utilizing Pharmacology Resources

Use a current edition of the *Physician's Desk Reference* (*PDR*) and look up the medication Valium. Answer the following questions:

1. What is its generic name? _____

2. What are the indications for its use? _____

_____

3. What does the symbol C-IV indicate? _____

4. Name three side effects/adverse reactions. _____

_____

5. How is it administered to patients? _____

Internet Exercises

Go to www.fda.gov and answer the following questions.

1. Search for a new medication that the FDA is investigating, currently monitoring, or has given approval for.

_____

2. What is this medication's precaution in regard to the pregnant patient? _____

_____

Go to www.osha.gov and describe the latest universal precautions protocol for sharps and needle sticks.

_____

_____

Go to www.nih.gov. What kind of health information can be found at this site?

_____

Go to www.nlm.nih.gov. What information can be found at this site? Select a current health news article and write a one-page report on the article's important points.

1. What is meant by an OTC medication?

    _____

2. According to the controlled substances classification schedule, what types of medications are considered C-I?

    _____

    _____

3. The study of genetic factors in predicting a medication's action in the body is called _____.

4. All of the following are found on a medication's label EXCEPT
    A. Pharmacy name
    B. Manufacturer's name
    C. Dosage strength
    D. Administration route

5. An example of a pharmacology resource that lists medication information is _____.

6. A narcotic is considered a/an
    A. OTC medication
    B. Controlled substance
    C. Nonprescription medication
    D. Low abuse-potential substance

7. Which federal agency within the U.S. Department of Labor has a mission to ensure safety of workers by establishing standards?
    A. DEA
    B. JCAHO
    C. CDC
    D. OSHA

8. The organization that evaluates and accredits health care institutions is
    A. DEA
    B. JCAHO
    C. CDE
    D. OSHA

9. In the phases of medication testing, which one is used on healthy volunteers to determine safe dosage levels?
    A. I
    B. II
    C. III
    D. IV

10. Which medication name is also called its trade name?
    A. Brand
    B. Chemical
    C. Generic
    D. Nonproprietary

CHAPTER REFERENCES

Kee JL, Hayes ER: Pharmacology: A Nursing Process Approach, 3rd ed. Philadelphia, WB Saunders, 2000.
Physician's Desk Reference, 59th ed. Montvale, NJ, Medical Economics, Inc, 2005.
Pickar G: Dosage Calculations, 6th ed. Albany, NY, Delmar, 1999.
www.cdc.gov
www.clinisphere.com
www.dea.gov
www.factsandcomparisons.com
www.fda.gov
www.jcaho.org
www.micromedex.com
www.ornl.gov/sci/techresources/human_genome/medicine/pharma.shtml
www.osha.gov

3 Pharmacology Math

After completing this chapter, you should be able to:
1. Convert civilian time to military time.
2. Define terminology, abbreviations, and symbols used in basic mathematics and measurement systems.
3. Use fractions in conversions and calculations.
4. Read and write decimals accurately.
5. Use decimals in conversions and calculations.
6. Convert between fractions and decimals.
7. Define percentages.
8. Convert between percentages and decimals and between percentages and fractions.
9. Define ratios and proportions.
10. Use ratios and proportions to solve problems.
11. Convert temperatures between Fahrenheit and Celsius scales.
12. Define the metric system of measurement and explain how it is used as the international standard.
13. Identify other systems of measurement and their medical applications.
14. Identify symbols of measurement and measurement equivalents.

CHAPTER OUTLINE

Learning the Language (Key Terms)

Using your textbook or a standard medical dictionary, look up and write the definition of each term.

1. Celsius scale: _____

2. Civilian time: _____

3. Decimal point: _____

4. Exponent: _____

5. Fahrenheit scale: _____

6. Fraction: _____

7. Metric system: _____

8. Military time: _____

9. Percent: _____

10. Proportion: _____

11. Ratio: _____

CHAPTER QUIZ

1. What is the military time for midnight? _____

2. What is the least common denominator for the fractions $\frac{1}{7}$ and $\frac{1}{8}$? _____

   _____

3. $4\frac{1}{4} \div \frac{1}{2} =$ _____ .

4. In the number 741.0059, the 5 is in the _____ position.

5. The value of 10^3 is _____ ?

6. In the order of operations, which is done LAST? _____
7. Place these decimal numbers in order beginning with the LARGEST number:
   (a) 0.00571 (b) 0.00057 (c) 0.0007

   _____

8. The measurement system also used as the international standard is the _____ .

9. 1 mm = _____ cc

10. 1 kg = _____ lbs

CHAPTER REFERENCES

Glazer EM, McConnell JW: Real-Life Math: Everyday Use of Mathematical Concepts. Westport, Conn, Greenwood, 2002.
Huettenmueller R: Algebra Demystified. New York, McGraw Hill, 2003.
Kee JL, Hayes ER: Pharmacology, 3rd ed. Philadelphia, WB Saunders, 2000.
Kee JL, Hayes ER: Study Guide for Pharmacology, 3rd ed. Philadelphia, WB Saunders, 2000.
McKeague CP: Intermediate Algebra: Functions & Graphs. Philadelphia, Harcourt Brace College Publishers, 1996.
McSharry P: Everyday Numbers. New York, Random House Reference, 2002.
Pickar GD: Dosage Calculations, 6th ed. Albany, NY, Delmar, 1999.
Ross D: Master Math: Basic Math and Pre-Algebra. Franklin Lakes, NJ, Career Press, 1996.
Slater J, Tobey J: Basic College Mathematics, 3rd ed. Upper Saddle River, NJ, Prentice Hall, 1998.
www.spacearchive.info/military.htm
www.usmilitary.about.com/od/jointservices/l/blmilitarytime.htm

4 Medication Administration

CHAPTER OBJECTIVES

After completing this chapter, you should be able to:
1. Describe the role of the surgical technologist in medication administration.
2. Explain the six "rights" of medication administration.
3. Describe the steps of medication identification.
4. Discuss aseptic techniques for delivery of medications to the sterile field.
5. State the procedure for labeling drugs on the sterile back table.
6. Identify supplies used in medication administration in surgery.

CHAPTER OUTLINE

    I. Surgical Technologist's Roles in Medication Administration
       A. Circulating Role
       B. Scrub Role
   II. The Six "Rights" of Medication Administration
       A. Right Drug
       B. Right Dose
       C. Right Route
       D. Right Patient
       E. Right Time
       F. Right Documentation
  III. Medication Identification
       A. All Team Members Responsible
       B. Identify and Document the Medication
       C. Label All Medications
  IV. Delivery to the Sterile Field
       A. Follow Principles of Asepsis
       B. Methods to Transfer Medications
       C. Containers for Medication Storage
    V. Medication Labeling on the Sterile Back Table
       A. Types of Labels
           1. Preprinted
           2. Blank labels
           3. Steri-Strips
       B. Precautions
  VI. Handling Medications
 VII. Supplies
       A. Syringes
       B. Hypodermic Needles
 VII. Advanced Practices for the Surgical First Assistant

CHAPTER CONTENT MASTERY

Learning the Language (Key Terms)

Using your textbook or a standard medical dictionary, look up and write the definition of each term.

1. Asepsis: _____

2. Carpule: _____

29

3. Contamination: _____

4. Diluent: _____

5. Hypersensitivity: _____

6. Reconstitute: _____

Chapter Review Questions

1. If you are currently in your clinical rotation, how is drug administration handled in surgery at your clinical facility?

_____

_____

2. Give examples of applications of the six "rights" of medication administration in surgery.

_____

_____

_____

_____

3. List the logical steps necessary to accurately identify drugs in surgery.

_____

_____

_____

4. Describe proper aseptic technique when delivering drugs to the sterile field.

_____

_____

5. If you are currently in your clinical rotation, what methods are used to label drugs on the sterile field at your clinical facility?

_____

_____

Critical Thinking

Scenario

It is 0725 and the patient has just been brought in to the operating room. The circulator is in a hurry because the patient has come into the room late and the surgeon is in the department. The circulator asks you to put the medication containers at the edge of the sterile back table so she can pour the solutions as soon as she has time and you can continue setting up for the procedure.

1. Is this safe practice? Justify your answer. _____

_____

2. List a better alternative to her request. _____

_____

Utilizing Pharmacology Resources

1. Investigate the legal parameters (as specified by your state) regarding medication administration. Write a summary of those parameters indicating statute and reference.

_____

_____

_____

2. Obtain a copy of a surgical technologist's job description from a local hospital. How is medication handling addressed? _____

_____

_____

3. Request a copy of the medication administration policy used in surgery at a clinical site. How are surgical technologists involved according to that policy? _____

_____

_____

Internet Exercises

1. Using your favorite search engine, look up the term *medication administration.*

a. How many "hits" did you get? _____

b. How many of the hits applied to surgical practice? _____

c. List two of the websites the search engine found for you.

_____

_____

d. Visit one of the websites you think is most reliable.

e. What was the most helpful information found on that site? _____

_____

2. Research the laws regarding medication administration in your state.

a. Where did you find information? (List the site.) _____
b. List the specific statutes that refer to medication administration in surgery.

_____

_____

1. Describe the role of a surgical technologist in medication administration in the circulating role.

   _____

2. Describe the role of a surgical technologist in medication administration in the first scrub role.

   _____

   _____

3. Explain one of the six "rights" of medication administration. _____

   _____

   _____

4. Describe the steps of medication identification. _____

   _____

5. List three aseptic techniques pertaining to delivery of medications to the sterile field.

   _____

   _____

   _____

6. State the procedure for labeling drugs on the sterile back table.

   _____

   _____

7. Identify two supplies used in medication administration in surgery.

   _____

   _____

ADVANCED PRACTICES CONTENT MASTERY

Learning the Language (Key Terms)

Using your textbook or a standard medical dictionary, look up and write the definition of each term.

1. Systemic effect:

   _____

2. Half-life:

   _____

Advanced Practices Chapter Review Questions

1. All of the following statements are true concerning patient effects from medication administration EXCEPT
   A. All medications have a systemic effect
   B. Topical medications affect only the localized area
   C. Liver function influences medication effects
   D. The time a medication is given influences its effect
2. When there is no state statute or federal law regulating an individual profession, who regulates health care workers in regard to medication administration?
   A. OSHA
   B. JCAHO
   C. Health care facilities
   D. Health department

3. The duration of a medication's effect is based on the medication's
   A. Dosage
   B. Strength
   C. Half-life
   D. Administration route

4. Explain why it is important to notify the anesthesia provider when a medication is administered at the sterile field.

   _____

   _____

5. Explain the pharmacologic principle known as the dose-time-effect relationship.

   _____

   _____

6. List the guidelines for administrating medications at the sterile field.

   _____

   _____

CHAPTER REFERENCES

Hopper T: Mosby's Pharmacy Technician Principles and Practice. St Louis, WB Saunders, 2004.
www.dea.gov
www.jcaho.org

ADVANCED PRACTICES CHAPTER REFERENCES

Gutierrez K: Pharmacotherapeutics: Clinical Decision-Making in Nursing. Philadelphia, WB Saunders, 1999.
Meeker M, Rothrock J: Alexander's Care of the Patient in Surgery, 12th ed. St Louis, Mosby, 2003.
Kee JL, Hayes ER: Pharmacology: A Nursing Process Approach, 3rd ed. Philadelphia, WB Saunders, 2000.

5 Antibiotics

CHAPTER OBJECTIVES

After completing this chapter, you should be able to:
1. Define terminology related to antimicrobial therapy.
2. Discuss the purpose of antibiotic therapy in surgery.
3. Describe various ways in which antimicrobials work.
4. Discuss antibiotic resistance.
5. List categories of antibiotics used in surgery and give examples of each.
6. Identify the category of various antibiotics.
7. Use drug resources to gather pertinent information on antibiotics.

CHAPTER OUTLINE

I. Microbiology Review
   A. Pathogenic Microorganisms
      1. Endogenous
      2. Exogenous
   B. Identification of Causative Microorganisms
      1. Culture and Sensitivity
         a. Aerobic Cultures
         b. Anaerobic Cultures
      2. Gram's Staining
   C. Prokaryotes
   D. Eukaryotes
II. Antimicrobial Action
   A. Mechanisms and Types
      1. Five Methods of Antimicrobial Action
      2. Bactericidal and Bacteriostatic Actions
   B. Antibiotic Resistance
      1. Penicillinase
      2. MRSA
      3. VRE
III. Antibiotic Agents
   A. Aminoglycosides
   B. Cephalosporins
   C. Macrolides
   D. Penicillins
   E. Tetracyclines
   F. Miscellaneous Antibiotics
IV. Advanced Practices for the Surgical First Assistant

CHAPTER CONTENT MASTERY

Learning the Language (Key Terms)

Using your textbook or a standard medical dictionary, look up and write the definition of each term.

1. Antibiotic resistance: _____

2. Bactericidal: _____

3. Bacteriostatic: _____

35

4. Culture and sensitivity (C&S): _____

5. Endogenous: _____

6. Eukaryotes: _____

7. Exogenous: _____

8. Gram's staining: _____

9. Morphology: _____

10. MRSA: _____

11. Nephrotoxicity: _____

12. Ototoxicity: _____

13. Polymicrobic infections: _____

14. Prokaryotes: _____

15. Prophylaxis: _____

16. Selective toxicity: _____

17. VRE: _____

Chapter Review Questions

1. What does MRSA stand for? VRE? Why are these important in surgery?

_____

_____

2. Why are antibiotics administered in surgery?

_____

3. Which test is used to identify the organism that causes TB?

_____

4. What does a C&S reveal?

_____

5. Why would a Gram's stain be ordered during surgery?

_____

6. How do antibiotics work?

_____

_____

7. What is the difference between bactericidal and bacteriostatic?

_____

8. Why is antimicrobial resistance a problem in surgery?

_____

9. How are antibiotics administered in surgery?

_____

10. Have you scrubbed or circulated in a procedure in which an antibiotic was administered? Which antibiotic was used? What category did the agent belong in? How was it administered?

_____

_____

_____

Critical Thinking

Scenario 1

Mrs. Chacon is a 55-year-old woman admitted to surgery for insertion of a venous access catheter. The chart indicates that she has an allergy to cefazolin (Ancef) and the preference card lists a standing order for cephalothin (Keflin) 1 gram mixed with 30 cc of NaCl for topical irrigation.

1. Is this medication order of concern? Explain why or why not.

_____

2. How should you handle this situation to ensure the patient's safety?

_____

Scenario 2

Mr. Fayed is a 33-year-old man who cut his hand while working in the garden 10 days ago. He was initially treated in the emergency room, where the wound was irrigated and closed. He was sent home with a prescription for piperacillin (Pipracil), which he has taken as instructed. The wound remains infected,

37

so he is admitted to surgery for incision and drainage of the wound. Swabs are taken for routine and fungal C&S, because the surgeon suspects the infectious agent may be a soil-based fungus.

1. How is a fungus different from bacteria?

2. Why wouldn't the antibiotic work on a fungal infection?

Visual Exercises

Indicate the major structures of a prokaryotic cell (Fig. 5–2A in the textbook) by labeling the drawing.
Word list: cell wall, DNA, nucleoid, plasma membrane, plasmid, ribosomes

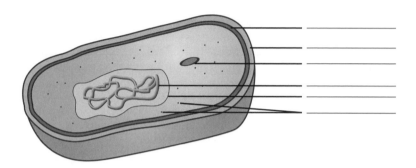

Indicate the major structures of a eukaryotic cell (Fig. 5–2B in the textbook) by labeling the drawing.
Word list: DNA, Golgi apparatus, mitochondrion, nuclear membrane, nucleolus, nucleus, plasma membrane, ribosomes, rough endoplasmic reticulum, smooth endoplasmic reticulum, vesicle

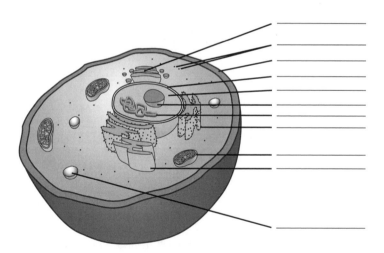

Utilizing Pharmacology Resources

1. Select an antibiotic that you or one of your family members has taken (or an assigned antibiotic). Complete a medication information sheet on the selected antibiotic using three different resources.
   a. Which source did you find most helpful and why?

   b. Which information was the most difficult to find?

Internet Exercises

1. Using your favorite search engine, look up an antibiotic listed in the textbook.

   a. How many "hits" did you get?_____

   b. How many of the hits applied to surgical practice?_____
   c. List two of the websites the search engine found for you.

   _____

   _____

   d. Visit one of the websites you think is most reliable.
   e. What was the most helpful information found on that site?

   _____

   _____

2. Using a different search engine, look up the same antibiotic.

   a. How many "hits" did you get? _____

   b. How many of the hits applied to surgical practice? _____
   c. List two different websites the search engine found for you. Do not use sites you used in the previous item.

   _____

   _____

   d. Visit one of the websites you think is most reliable.
   e. What was the most helpful information found on that site?

   _____

   _____

3. Select an antibiotic from each major category and enter each one in a search engine to find the pharmaceutical manufacturer for each antibiotic.
   a. Where did you find information? (List the site.)

   _____

   b. Does any manufacturer appear more frequently? Less frequently?

   _____

   _____

1. Define the term *bactericidal*.

_____

2. All of the following are ways antimicrobials work EXCEPT
   A. Inhibit cell-wall synthesis
   B. Interfere with cell metabolism
   C. Inhibit production of nucleic acids (RNA or DNA)
   D. Interfere with function of endoplasmic reticulum
3. Eukaryotic cells differ from prokaryotic cells in that they lack a
   A. Cell wall
   B. Cytoplasm
   C. Golgi complex
   D. True nucleus
4. Penicillinase is a/an
   A. Acid
   B. Antibiotic
   C. Enzyme
   D. Nucleic acid
5. Discuss two aspects of antibiotic resistance.

_____

_____

_____

6. Gentamicin (Garamycin) is in which of the following categories of antibiotics?
   A. Aminoglycoside
   B. Cephalosporin
   C. Macrolide
   D. Tetracycline
7. Cefixime (Suprax) is in which of the following categories of antibiotics?
   A. Aminoglycoside
   B. Cephalosporin
   C. Macrolide
   D. Tetracycline
8. List two resources used to gather pertinent information on antibiotics.

_____

_____

_____

ADVANCED PRACTICES CONTENT MASTERY

Learning the Language (Key Terms)
Using your textbook or a standard medical dictionary, look up and write the definition of each term.
1. Peak and trough:

_____

2. Sepsis:

_____

3. SSI:

_____

Advanced Practices Chapter Review Questions

1. List three factors to consider when choosing an appropriate antibiotic.

   a. _____

   b. _____

   c. _____

2. The time when a medication is at the highest plasma concentration is referred to as the

   _____ .

3. The decay and putrefaction of living tissue from an overwhelming infection is called
   A. Dehydration
   B. Sepsis
   C. Sciatica
   D. Necrosis

4. How long before a surgical procedure should preoperative prophylactic antibiotics be administered?
   A. 10 minutes
   B. 30 minutes
   C. 1 hour
   D. 2 hours

5. An antibiotic commonly used within the sterile field is _____ .

CHAPTER REFERENCES

Baron E, Chang R, Howard D, et al: Medical Microbiology a Short Course. New York, Wiley-Liss, 1994.
Bergquist L, Pogosian B: Microbiology Principles and Health Science Applications. Philadelphia, WB Saunders, 2000.
Hopper T: Mosby's Pharmacy Technician Principles and Practice. St Louis, WB Saunders, 2004.
Price P, Frey K: Microbiology for Surgical Technologists. Clifton Park, NY, Thomson Delmar Learning, 2003.
Saeb-Parsy K, Assomull RG, Khan FZ, et al: Instant Pharmacology. Chichester, England, Wiley and Sons, 1999.
www.cdc.gov/drugresistance/community/
www.fda.gov/fdac/features/795_antibio.html
www.fda.gov/oc/opacom/hottopics/anti_resist.html
helios.bto.ed.ac.uk/bto/microbes/penicill.htm
www.hhmi.org/biointeractive/Antibiotics_Attack/frameset.html
www.howstuffworks.com/question88.htm
micro.magnet.fsu.edu/micro/gallery/pharm/antibiotic/antibiotic.html
www.molbio.princeton.edu/courses/mb427/2001/projects/02/antibiotics.htm
www.nlm.nih.gov/medlineplus/antibiotics.html
www.umm.edu/altmed/ConsDrugs/DrugCats/Antibiotics.html
users.rcn.com/jkimball.ma.ultranet/BiologyPages/A/Antibiotics.html

ADVANCED PRACTICES CHAPTER REFERENCES

Gutierrez K: Pharmacotherapeutics: Clinical Decision-Making in Nursing, Philadelphia, WB Saunders, 1999.

6 Diagnostic Agents

CHAPTER OBJECTIVES

After completing this chapter, you should be able to:
1. Define contrast media, dyes, and staining agents.
2. Give examples of contrast media and how each is used in radiographic studies in surgery.
3. Give examples of dyes and how each is used in surgical procedures.
4. Give examples of staining agents and how each is used in surgical procedures.

CHAPTER OUTLINE

   I. Contrast Media
     A. Definitions
     B. Examples and Uses
       1. Omnipaque
       2. Hypaque
       3. Visipaque
       4. Isovue
  II. Dyes
     A. Definitions
     B. Examples and Uses
       1. Methylene Blue
       2. Isosulfan Blue
       3. Indigo Carmine
       4. Gentian Violet
 III. Staining Agents
     A. Definitions
     B. Examples and Uses
       1. Lugol's Solution
       2. Acetic Acid
 IV. Advanced Practices for the Surgical First Assistant

CHAPTER CONTENT MASTERY

Learning the Language (Key Terms)
Using your textbook or a standard medical dictionary, look up and write the definition of each term.

1. Contraindicated: _____

2. Contrast media: _____

3. Dye: _____

4. Hypersensitivity: _____

5. Radiopaque: _____

6. Staining agent: _____

Chapter Review Questions

1. What is the difference between contrast media and dyes?_____

_____

2. Why should contrast media be labeled on the sterile back table?_____

_____

3. How does Isosulfan blue (Lymphazurin) help the surgeon find the sentinel node?

_____

4. Why should the patient's medical history for allergies be considered before contrast media are

administered?_____

_____

5. How is methylene blue used in tubal dye studies (TDS)?_____

_____

Critical Thinking

1. List two ways to label your contrast media on the back table._____

_____

_____

2. Explain the importance of sentinel lymph node biopsy for breast cancer diagnosis.

_____

_____

3. How do surgeons at clinical facilities mark incision sites?

_____

_____

4. Name a procedure that uses methylene blue placed into the bladder.

_____

_____

Scenario

Nancy Cho is scheduled for a cholecystectomy and a common bile duct exploration. Her diagnosis is cholecystitis and cholelithiasis. You have Hypaque 50% and normal saline 50 cc on the back table.

1. The patient's chart should be checked for allergies. What allergy in particular would impact her

cholangiogram?_____

_____

2. Both Hypaque and normal saline are drawn up into 30 cc syringes. How are they properly identified

on the field?_____

_____

44

Chapter **6** **Diagnostic Agents**

3. Which solution is injected first? Why? _____

_____

4. Where are these solutions injected for the procedure? _____

_____

_____

Utilizing Pharmacology Resources

Use the Internet as a pharmacology resource. Go to www.medlineplus.com and look under the topic "drug information" for Lugol's solution. Answer the following questions.

1. What is its category? _____

2. What is its description? _____

_____

3. List five side effects of this medication. _____

_____

_____

_____

4. With what national agency is MedlinePlus associated? _____

_____

Internet Exercises

Do an Internet search for gentian violet. What uses can be found for this dye?

_____

_____

CHAPTER QUIZ

1. Contrast are what type of chemicals?
   A. Staining
   B. Radiopaque
   C. Topical
   D. Radiotransparent
2. What agents are used to identify abnormal cells, especially on the cervix?
   A. Contrast media
   B. Dyes
   C. Staining agents
   D. Antifungals
3. What iodine mixture is used in a Schiller's test?
   A. Lugol's solution
   B. Lymphazurin
   C. Methylene blue
   D. Omnipaque

4. _____ is often used in surgery for an operative cholangiogram.

5. _____ are solutions that mark tissue for skin incisions.
6. The dye used in sentinel node biopsy procedures is
   A. Omnipaque
   B. Hypaque
   C. Isovue
   D. Lymphazurin
7. Most contrast media solutions contain
   A. Iodine
   B. Potassium
   C. Vinegar
   D. Chloride

8. If a contrast media is contraindicated, it means it is _____.
9. What is used to demonstrate blockages or abnormalities in the vascular system?
   A. Myelography
   B. Urography
   C. Cholangiography
   D. Angiography

10. _____ is used to test the patency of the fallopian tubes.

ADVANCED PRACTICES CONTENT MASTERY

Learning the Language (Key Terms)

Using your textbook or a standard medical dictionary, look up and write the definition of each term.

1. ARF:_____

2. Diaphoresis:_____

3. Hydration:_____

4. Iodinated: _____

5. Nephrotoxicity: _____

6. Urticaria: _____

Advanced Practices Chapter Review Questions

1. Which route of administration for iodinated contrast media is more likely to cause an adverse reaction?
   A. Oral
   B. Intravascular
   C. Extravascular
   D. Rectal

2. Name three risk factors that may contribute to acute renal failure after administration of contrast media.

   _____   _____   _____

3. Which is the current treatment to reduce nephrotoxicity after the administration of contrast media?
   A. Antibiotic therapy
   B. Administration of a vasodilator
   C. Hydration
   D. Dehydration

4. Name three symptoms of an adverse reaction to contrast media.

   _____   _____   _____

5. A new ultrasonic diagnostic contrast media used to study the heart consists of millions of

   _____ .

CHAPTER REFERENCES

D'Amours A: Sentinel lymph node biopsy and lymphoscintigraphy. Surg Technologist 35:1, 2003.
Henry MM, Thompson JN: Clinical Surgery. Philadelphia, WB Saunders, 2001.
Phillips N: Berry and Kohn's Operating Room Technique, 10th ed. St Louis, Mosby, 2004.
Townsend CM Jr: Sabiston Textbook of Surgery, 16th ed. Philadelphia, WB Saunders, 2001.
www.amershamhealth.com/medcyclopedia
www.asccp.org/practice
www.com/cons/lugol_s_solution.html
www.medsafe.govt.nz/profs/datasheet/I/Isovueinj.htm
www.nlm.nih.gov/medlineplus/druginfo/uspdi/202259.html
www.nlm.nih.gov/medlineplus/druginfo/uspdi/202703.html
www.rxlist.com/cgi/generic3/indocarmine.htm
www.rxmed.com

ADVANCED PRACTICES CHAPTER REFERENCES

archfami/ama-assn.org/cgi/reprint/9/8/748.pdf
www.biz.yahoo.com/prNews/040909/sfth058_1.html
www.emedicine.com/radio/topic864.htm
www.evidenttech.com/why_nano/why_nano.php
www.medicinenet.com/methylprednisolone/article/htm
www.medreviews.com/pdfs/articles/RICM_2Suppl_S9/pdf
www.nlm.nih.gov/medlineplus/druginfo/medmaster/a682866.html
www.rxlist.com/cgi/generic/methprd.htm
www.rxlist.com/cgi/generic/cimet/htm

7 | Diuretics

CHAPTER OBJECTIVES

After completing this chapter, you should be able to:
1. State the general purpose of a diuretic.
2. Describe the physiology of the kidney.
3. Identify anatomic structures of the nephron.
4. List diseases that use diuretics for management.
5. Describe the impact of long-term diuretic therapy on the patient about to undergo a surgical procedure.
6. Discuss the type of patient who may come to surgery on long-term diuretic therapy.
7. Differentiate between the purposes for long-term and short-term use of diuretics.
8. List the two most common diuretics administered intraoperatively and their purpose.

CHAPTER OUTLINE

I. Definition of Diuretics
   A. Management of Medical Conditions
   B. Excretion of Electrolytes
   C. Effects on the Surgical Patient
II. Review of Renal Physiology
   A. Filtering of Blood
   B. Removal of Substances from the Blood
      1. Excess Water
      2. Solutes
III. Diuretics
   A. Loop Diuretics
   B. Thiazide Diuretics
   C. Potassium-Sparing Diuretics
   D. Carbonic Anhydrase Inhibitors
   E. Osmotic Diuretics
IV. Advanced Practices for the Surgical First Assistant

CHAPTER CONTENT MASTERY

Learning the Language (Key Terms)

Using your textbook or a standard medical dictionary, look up and write the definition of each term.

1. CHF: _____

2. Creatinine: _____

3. Diuresis: _____

4. Diuretic: _____

5. Dysrhythmia: _____

6. Electrolyte: _____

49

7. Glaucoma: _____

8. Homeostasis: _____

9. Hyperkalemia: _____

10. Hypertension: _____

11. Hypokalemia: _____

12. Nephron: _____

Chapter Review Questions

1. How does the nephron work to eliminate waste products and excess water?

_____

2. How do diuretics work?_____

_____

3. Which structures of the nephron are affected by diuretics?_____

_____

4. Why would a diuretic be prescribed for long-term use?_____

_____

5. What is a common adverse effect of long-term diuretic therapy on a patient? How does that condition

   impact the administration of a general anesthetic?_____

_____

6. What type of patient may come to surgery on long-term diuretic therapy?_____

_____

7. Why are diuretics used intraoperatively?_____

_____

8. Which diuretics are used intraoperatively?_____

_____

Critical Thinking

Scenario 1

Mrs. Hernandez is an 85-year-old woman admitted to surgery for insertion of a hip prosthesis to treat a hip fracture. The surgical technologist assigned to transport the patient to the preoperative holding area performed a routine review of the patient's medical chart in the emergency department. The medical chart indicates that Mrs. Hernandez is being treated for chronic hypertension.

1. Knowing that she has a concurrent diagnosis of hypertension, which additional related items should be checked on her chart?

_____

_____

2. How might this situation affect the preparations going on in the surgery department?

_____

3. What action(s) should the surgical technologist take prior to bringing the patient to preoperative holding?

_____

_____

Scenario 2

Mr. Van Nguyen is a 47-year-old man admitted to surgery for repair of a retinal detachment under general anesthesia.

1. Which diuretic may be administered intraoperatively?_____

2. The circulator should check the preference card for a standing order for what preoperative preparation

   specific to this situation?_____

_____

51

Visual Exercises

Indicate the structures of a nephron (Fig. 7–1 in the textbook) by labeling the drawing.

Word list: afferent arteriole, ascending loop, collecting duct, descending loop, distal convoluted tubule, efferent arteriole, glomerular (Bowman's) capsule, glomerulus, loop of the nephron, proximal convoluted tubule

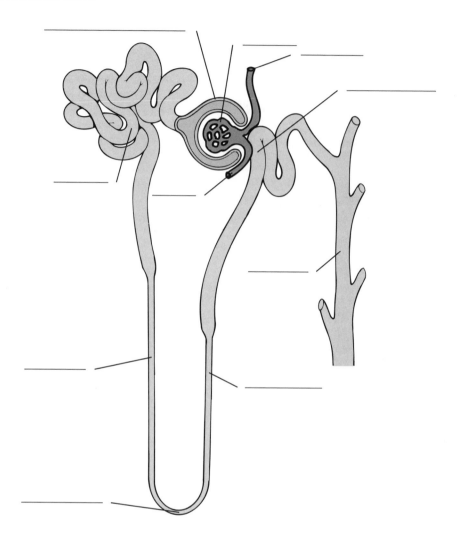

Utilizing Pharmacology Resources

1. Complete a medication information sheet on furosemide (Lasix) using two different resources.

   a. Which source did you find most helpful and why?_____

   _____

   b. What information was the most difficult to find?_____

   _____

2. Complete a medication information sheet on mannitol (Osmitrol) using two different resources than those used in the previous exercise.

   a. Which source did you find most helpful and why? _____

   _____

   b. What information was the most difficult to find?_____

   _____

Internet Exercises

1. Using your favorite search engine, look up congestive heart failure.

   a. How many "hits" did you get?_____

   b. List two of the websites the search engine found for you._____

   _____

   _____

   c. Visit one of the websites you think is most reliable.

   d. What was the most helpful information found on that site?_____

   _____

   e. How will the information you learned help you in clinical practice?_____

   _____

2. Using a different search engine, look up either furosemide or mannitol.

   a. How many "hits" did you get? _____

   b. How many of the hits applied to surgical practice?_____

   c. List two different websites the search engine found for you. Do not use sites you used in the previous exercise.

   _____

   _____

   d. Visit one of the websites you think is most reliable.

   e. What was the most helpful information found on that site?_____

   _____

   _____

1. Define the term *diuretic*.

2. State the general purpose of a diuretic._____

3. Which of the following processes takes place in the glomerular capsule?
   A. Filtration
   B. Reabsorption
   C. Secretion
   D. Transformation

4. All of the following diseases use diuretics for management EXCEPT
   A. Congestive heart failure
   B. Glaucoma
   C. Hyperlipidemia
   D. Hypertension

5. The surgical patient who has been on long term diuretic therapy may also have the related condition of
   A. Hypercalcemia
   B. Hypocalcemia
   C. Hyperkalemia
   D. Hypokalemia

6. Which of the following patients may most likely come to surgery on diuretics?
   A. 32-year-old woman with diabetes
   B. 47-year-old man with cholecystitis
   C. 62-year-old woman with a fractured wrist
   D. 85-year-old man with hypotension

7. State the purpose of long-term diuretic therapy._____

8. State the purpose of short-term diuretic therapy._____

9. List the two most common diuretics administered in surgery._____

ADVANCED PRACTICES CONTENT MASTERY

Learning the Language (Key Terms)

Using your textbook or a standard medical dictionary, look up and write the definition of each term.

1. Diuresis:

2. Hypokalemia:

Advanced Practices Chapter Review Questions

1. The term to describe a depletion of potassium in the blood serum is
   A. Hypovolemia
   B. Hypocalcemia
   C. Hypothermia
   D. Hypokalemia

2. Normal level of potassium in blood serum is _____ mEq/L.

3. Describe the treatment for chronic and acute hypokalemia. _____

_____

4. Which category of medications causes the highest rate of potassium depletion?
   A. Antibiotics
   B. Analgesics
   C. Diuretics
   D. Steroids

5. Name two food sources that are high in potassium. _____

_____

CHAPTER REFERENCES

Duke J: Anesthesia Secrets, 2nd ed. Philadelphia, Hanley and Belfus, 2000.
Hopper T: Mosby's Pharmacy Technician Principles and Practice. St Louis, WB Saunders, 2004.
Nagelhout J, Zaglaniczny K, Haglund V: Handbook of Nurse Anesthesia, 2nd ed. Philadelphia, WB Saunders, 2001.
Saeb-Parsy K, Assomull RG, Khan FZ, et al: Instant Pharmacology. Chichester, England, Wiley and Sons, 1999.
Simpson P, Popat M: Understanding Anaesthesia, 4th ed. Edinburgh, Butterworth Heineman, 2002.
lysine.pharm.utah.edu/netpharm/netpharm_00/notes/diuretics.html
www.bupa.co.uk/health_information/html/medicine/loop_diuretics.html
www.mayoclinic.com/printinvoker.cfm?objectid=E7492D61-D3D0-4624-9EBDA3A85E08B557
www.nlm.nih.gov/medlineplus/druginfo/uspdi/202208.html
www.outlinemed.com/demo/nephrol/7640.htm
www.preceptor.com/CrsCardiology/car/diuretic.htm
www.uspharmacist.com/oldformat.asp?url=newlook/files/Feat/ACF2EDE.cfm&pub_id=8&article_id=24

ADVANCED PRACTICES CHAPTER REFERENCES

Agarwal A, Wingo CS: Treatment of hypokalemia. N Engl J Med 340:154, 1999.
Cameron JL: Current Surgical Therapy. St Louis, Mosby, 2001.
Gennari JF: Hypokalemia. N Engl J Med 339:451, 1998.
Gutierrez K: Pharmacotherapeutics: Clinical Decision-Making in Nursing. Philadelphia, WB Saunders, 1999.
Kee JL, Hayes ER: Pharmacology: A Nursing Process Approach, 4th ed. Philadelphia, WB Saunders, 2003.
www.healthyhearts.com/diuretic.htm
www.krispin.com/potassm.html
www.nlm.nih.gov/medlineplus/druginfo/uspdi/202208.html

8 Hormones

CHAPTER OBJECTIVES

After completing this chapter, you should be able to:
1. Define terminology related to the endocrine system.
2. List endocrine glands and hormones secreted by each.
3. State the purpose for administration of each hormone.
4. Describe medical and surgical uses for hormones.
5. List hormones that may be administered from the sterile field.
6. List procedures that may require administration of hormones from the sterile field.

CHAPTER OUTLINE

I. Endocrine System Review
   A. Chemical Messengers Called Hormones
   B. Regulation of Growth, Development, Reproduction, and Homeostasis
II. Endocrine Glands
   A. Pituitary Gland
      1. Adenohypophysis
         a. Growth Hormone (GH)
         b. Thyroid-Stimulating Hormone (TSH)
         c. Adrenocorticotropic Hormone (ACTH)
         d. Follicle-Stimulating Hormone (FSH)
         e. Luteinizing Hormone (LH)
         f. Prolactin (PRL)
      2. Neurohypophysis
         a. Oxytoxin
         b. Antidiuretic Hormone (ADH)
   B. Thyroid Gland
      1. Thyroxine (T-4)
      2. Triiodothyronine (T-3)
      3. Calcitonin
   C. Parathyroid Glands
   D. Adrenal Glands
      1. Medulla
         a. Epinephrine
         b. Norepinephrine
      2. Cortex
         a. Glucocorticoids
         b. Mineralocorticoids
   E. Pancreas
      1. Endocrine Gland
         a. Insulin
         b. Glucagon
      2. Exocrine Gland
   F. Ovaries
      1. Estrogen
      2. Progesterone
   G. Testes
III. Advanced Practices for the Surgical First Assistant

Learning the Language (Key Terms)

Using your textbook or a standard medical dictionary, look up and write the definition of each term.

1. Amenorrhea: _____

2. Androgen: _____

3. Dysmenorrhea: _____

4. Endometriosis: _____

5. Fibrocystic disease of the breast: _____

6. Fight-or-flight response: _____

7. Hyperparathyroidism: _____

8. Hyperthyroidism: _____

9. Hypoglycemic drugs: _____

10. Hypogonadism: _____

11. Hypoparathyroidism: _____

12. Hypothyroidism: _____

13. Menopause: _____

14. Osteoporosis: _____

15. Palliatives: _____

16. Recombinant DNA technology: _____

Chapter Review Questions

1. For which surgical procedure is oxytoxin used?_____

_____

2. What are the hormones produced by the adenohypophysis?_____

_____

3. What are the hormones produced by the neurohypophysis?_____

_____

4. Describe recombinant DNA technology in hormone synthesis._____

_____

_____

5. How are steroids administered to the medical patient? The surgical patient?_____

_____

_____

6. What portion of the pancreas produces hormones?_____

_____

7. Why would a male receive a female hormone? A female receive a male hormone?_____

_____

8. What surgical procedures might involve injection of steroids?_____

_____

Critical Thinking

1. Can you think of other medications that are given for palliative purposes?_____

_____

2. What are the strengths of epinephrine normally encountered in the surgical setting?

_____

Scenario

Joseph Goldstein is a 55-year-old man scheduled for a total thyroidectomy. His diagnosis is carcinoma of the thyroid gland. Answer the following questions as they relate to Mr. Goldstein's procedure.

1. What other endocrine glands would be involved in this procedure?_____

_____

2. Where are these other glands located?_____

_____

3. How will the removal of the thyroid and these other glands affect the patient postoperatively?

_____

4. What can be done to correct any imbalances caused by removing the thyroid glands?

_____

Visual Exercises

Label the drawing (Fig. 8–1 in the textbook) with the endocrine glands and list the hormone(s) each secretes.

  Word list: adrenal glands, digestive tract, heart, hypothalamus, kidney, ovaries, pancreas, parathyroid glands, pineal gland, pituitary gland, testes, thymus gland, thyroid gland

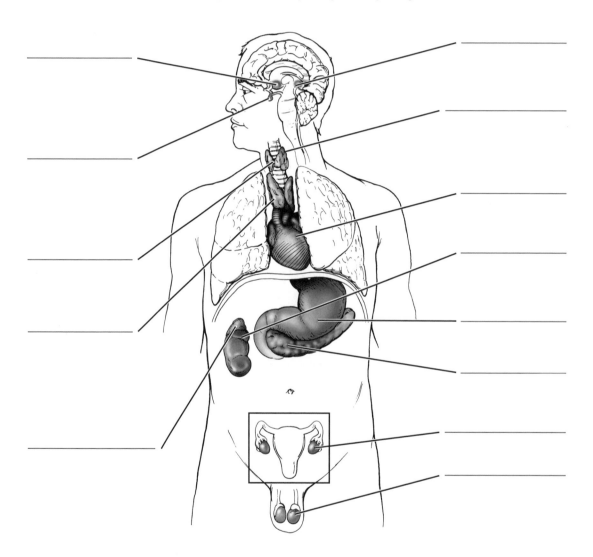

Utilizing Pharmacology Resources

Using *Mosby's Drug Consult,* look up Hormones/Hormone Modifiers. Under this topic, look up oxytocin and answer the following questions.

1. What is its brand name?_____

2. How is it administered to the patient?_____

3. What is its indication for use?_____

60

4. List three adverse reactions from this medication.

_____

_____

Internet Exercises

Consult *Mosby's Drug Consult* or do an Internet search to compare Pitocin and Pitressin. Answer the following questions for both medications.

1. What are the indications?

2. What are the side effects/adverse reactions?

_____

3. What are the generic names?

_____

1. Which endocrine gland is known as the master gland?_____

   _____

2. Hormones help regulate all of the following body functions EXCEPT
   A. Internal chemical balance
   B. Growth and development
   C. Reproduction
   D. Digestion
3. Which gland(s) sets the rate of body metabolism?
   A. Thyroid
   B. Parathyroid
   C. Adrenal
   D. Ovaries
4. What is produced by the adrenal medulla and used with local anesthetics to prolong their effect?
   A. Insulin
   B. Epinephrine
   C. Pitocin
   D. Glucose
5. Steroids are produced by the
   A. Parathyroid glands
   B. Adrenal medulla
   C. Adrenal cortex
   D. Testes
6. The gland that is both endocrine and exocrine is the
   A. Pituitary
   B. Pancreas
   C. Parathyroid
   D. Pineal
7. Insulin is produced in the
   A. Adrenal cortex
   B. Adrenal medulla
   C. Anterior pituitary
   D. Isles of Langerhans
8. Inadequate amounts of parathyroid hormone result in
   A. Hyperparathyroidism
   B. Hypoparathyroidism
   C. Hyperthyroidism
   D. Hypothyroidism
9. What hormone stimulates uterine contractions?
   A. Cortisol
   B. Corticosterone
   C. Estrogen
   D. Oxytoxin
10. Medications given to relieve symptoms but that do not cure the disease are called _____.

ADVANCED PRACTICES CONTENT MASTERY

Learning the Language (Key Terms)

Using your textbook or a standard medical dictionary, look up and write the definition of each term.

1. Euthyroid: _____

2. Hypercalcemia: _____

3. Hypocalcemia: _____

Advanced Practices Chapter Review Questions

1. Which two endocrine glands are most commonly affected by a disorder or disease?

   _____   _____

2. At the time of any thyroid surgery, it is best for the patient to be
   A. Hyperthyroid
   B. Hypothyroid
   C. Euthyroid
   D. Any of the above

3. List three symptoms of thyroid storm.

   _____   _____   _____

4. Which is the most common disorder of the endocrine system that may cause a patient's blood calcium to be elevated?
   A. Hyperthyroidism
   B. Hyperparathyroidism
   C. Hypothyroidism
   D. Hypoparathyroidism

5. Describe the common causes of primary and secondary hyperparathyroidism.

   _____

6. What is the most common cause of hypoparathyroidism?_____

   _____

CHAPTER REFERENCES

Khatri VP, Asensio JA: Operative Surgery Manual. Philadelphia, WB Saunders, 2003.
Martini FH: Fundamentals of Anatomy and Physiology, 5th ed. Upper Saddle River, NJ, Prentice Hall, 2001.
Rothrock J: Alexander's Care of the Patient in Surgery, 12th ed. St Louis, Mosby, 2003.
www.accessexcellence.org/AB/IE/Speaking_Language_rDNA.html
www.nigms.nih.gov/news/science_ed/definitn/recomb.html
www.sciencemag.org/feature/e-market/benchtop/ddbt_31904.shl

ADVANCED PRACTICES CHAPTER REFERENCES

Banks P, Kraybill W: Pathology for the Surgeon. Philadelphia, WB Saunders, 1996.
Cameron JL: Current Surgical Therapy. St Louis, Mosby, 2001.
Gutierrez K: Pharmacotherapeutics: Clinical Decision-Making in Nursing. Philadelphia, WB Saunders, 1999.
Kee JL, Hayes ER: Pharmacology: A Nursing Process Approach. Philadelphia, WB Saunders, 2003.
Khatri VP, Asensio JA: Operative Surgery Manual. Philadelphia, WB Saunders, 2003.
Merli GJ, Weitz HH: Medical Management of the Surgical Patient. Philadelphia, WB Saunders, 1992.
cpmcnet.columbia.edu/dept/thyroid/parasurgHP.html
www.emedicine.com/med/topic917.htm
www.emedicine.com/ped/byname/thyroid-storm.htm
www.endocrineweb.com/function.html
www.endocrineweb.com/whatisendo.html
www.MERCK.com/pubs/mmanual/section2/chapter8/8e.htm
www.nlm.nih.gov/medlineplus/print/druginfo/medmaster/a682465.html
www.pathologyoutlines.com/parathyroidpf.html
www.thyroidmanager.org/Chapter12/12-text.htm
www.yourmedicalsource.com/library/hyperthyroidism/HYE_surgery.html

9 Medications That Affect Coagulation

CHAPTER OBJECTIVES

After completing this chapter, you should be able to:
1. Define terms related to blood coagulation and medications that affect coagulation.
2. Describe the physiology of blood clot formation.
3. List agents that affect coagulation by category.
4. Identify the category of various agents that affect coagulation.
5. State the purpose of each category of medications that affect coagulation.
6. Describe the action of medications that affect coagulation.
7. List uses, routes of administration, side effects, and contraindications for agents that affect coagulation.
8. Describe the impact of preoperative oral anticoagulant therapy on the surgical patient.
9. List examples of surgical procedures in which agents that affect coagulation may be administered.
10. Compare and contrast administration route, onset of action, antagonist, and purpose of parenteral and oral anticoagulants.
11. List the administration route for each medication that affects coagulation.

CHAPTER OUTLINE

   I. Introduction to the Coagulation Process
  II. Physiology of Clot Formation
 III. Coagulants
    A. Hemostatics
       1. Absorbable Gelatin
       2. Microfibrillar Collagen Hemostat
       3. Oxidized Cellulose
       4. Absorbable Collagen Sponge
       5. Thrombin
       6. Bone Wax
       7. Chemical Hemostatics
    B. Systemic Coagulants
       1. Calcium Salts
       2. Vitamin K
       3. Blood Coagulation Factors
  IV. Anticoagulants
    A. Parenteral Anticoagulants
    B. Oral Anticoagulants
    C. Thrombolytics
   V. Advanced Practices for the Surgical First Assistant

CHAPTER CONTENT MASTERY

Learning the Language (Key Terms)

Using your textbook or a standard medical dictionary, look up and write the definition of each term.

1. Anticoagulants: _____

2. Coagulants: _____

3. Coagulation (clotting) factors: _____

4. Hemostatics: _____

65

5. Parenteral: _____

6. Platelet aggregation: _____

7. Systemic: _____

8. Thrombolytics (fibrinolytics): _____

9. Thrombosis: _____

Chapter Review Questions

1. If you are in your clinical rotation, which hemostatic agents are used most frequently in your clinical facility? In which procedures? _____

_____

2. Why are hemostatics used? _____

3. What are systemic coagulants used for? Can you name some? _____

4. Name three surgical procedures that usually require heparin ready on the back table. In which strengths? _____

5. How does oral anticoagulant therapy affect the patient about to undergo a surgical procedure?

_____

6. Why are thrombolytics administered? _____

Critical Thinking

Scenario 1

You are scrubbed for a repair of an abdominal aortic aneurysm. The preference card indicates that Dr. Fromm wants 5000 units of heparin in 500 mL of saline for topical irrigation. The circulator can only find carpules containing 10,000 units/mL of heparin.

1. What is one solution to this problem?

_____

2. What is another solution to this problem?

_____

Scenario 2

Mr. Davis is a 67-year-old man admitted to surgery for an immediate laparoscopic cholecystectomy for acute cholecystitis. Review of his medical chart reveals that he is on coumadin (Warfarin).

1. What complications do you expect to see during this procedure?

_____

2. What additional supplies should you bring in the room in preparation for these complications?

_____

3. What actions may be taken during surgery to treat these complications?

_____

_____

Utilizing Pharmacology Resources

1. Complete a medication information sheet on heparin using two different resources.

   a. Which source did you find most helpful and why? _____

   b. Which information was the most difficult to find? _____

Internet Exercises

1. Using a search engine you've never tried before, look up the drug heparin.

   a. How many "hits" did you get? _____

   b. List two of the websites the search engine found for you. _____

      _____

   c. Visit one of the websites you think is most reliable.
   d. What was the most helpful information found on that site?

      _____

   e. How will the information you learned help you in clinical practice?

      _____

2. Using the same search engine, look up one type of hemostatic agent by brand name.

   a. How many "hits" did you get? _____
   b. List two different websites the search engine found for you. Do not use sites you used in the previous exercise.

      _____

      _____

   c. Visit one of the websites you think is most reliable.
   d. What was the most helpful information found on that site?

      _____

3. Using your favorite search engine, attempt to locate a website that provides visual images of the blood coagulation process. Then go to
   http://tollefsen.wustl.edu/projects/coagulation/coagulation.html

   a. Which site did you prefer? _____

   b. Which site was more helpful and why? _____

1. Define the term *parenteral*.

_____

2. Which of the following coagulation pathways is activated due to trauma?
   A. Extrinsic
   B. Intrinsic
3. Which of the following is a systemic coagulant?
   A. Heparin sodium
   B. Phytonadione (Konakion)
   C. Thrombin
   D. Warfarin (Coumadin)
4. Oxidized cellulose is a/an
   A. Anticoagulant
   B. Hemostatic
   C. Systemic coagulant
   D. Thrombolytic
5. State the purpose of a hemostatic agent.

_____

6. Describe the action of heparin.

_____

7. Calcium salts are contraindicated in patients with a history of
   A. Congestive heart failure
   B. Diabetes
   C. Hypertension
   D. Malignant hyperthermia
8. Describe the impact of preoperative oral anticoagulant therapy on the surgical patient.

_____

_____

9. List a specific surgical procedure in which heparin may be administered from the back table.

_____

10. The antagonist for warfarin (Coumadin) is
    A. Acetylsalicylic acid
    B. Factor IX complex
    C. Protamine sulfate
    D. Vitamin K

ADVANCED PRACTICES CONTENT MASTERY

Learning the Language (Key Terms)

Using your textbook or a standard medical dictionary, look up and write the definition of each term.

1. Anticoagulation therapy: _____

2. INR: _____

3. PT: _____

1. Why is it necessary for patients on anticoagulation therapy to be closely monitored?

   _____

2. What type of procedures may require short-term anticoagulation therapy?

   _____

3. What condition is treated with short-term anticoagulation therapy postoperatively?

   _____

   _____

4. The most common medication used for short-term anticoagulation is _____ and its normal dosage is _____ u/kg of patient weight.

5. One indication for long-term anticoagulation therapy is _____.

6. How does Warfarin produce its anticoagulation effect? _____

7. List three oral anticoagulant medications and an indication for each.

   _____

   _____

   _____

   _____

CHAPTER REFERENCES

Duke J: Anesthesia Secrets, 2nd ed. Philadelphia, Hanley and Belfus, 2000.
Hopper T: Mosby's Pharmacy Technician Principles and Practice. St Louis, WB Saunders, 2004.
Nagelhout J, Zaglaniczny K, Haglund V: Handbook of Nurse Anesthesia, 2nd ed. Philadelphia, WB Saunders, 2001.
Saeb-Parsy K, Assomull RG, Khan FZ, et al: Instant Pharmacology. Chichester, England, Wiley and Sons, 1999.
Simpson P, Popat M: Understanding Anesthesia, 4th ed. Edinburgh, Butterworth Heinemann, 2002.
web.indstate.edu/thcme/mwking/blood-coagulation.html
www.bleedingweb.com/
www.coagulation-factors.com/
www.davol.com/HTMLFiles/Hemostasis/HemostasisProducts1.html
www.gene.com/gene/products/information/cardiovascular/activase/insert.jsp
www.jnjgateway.com/home.jhtml?page=menu&nodekey=/Prod_Info/Type/Surgical_Wound_Care/Hemostasis
www.lovenox.com/
www.medicinenet.com/warfarin/article.htm
www.merck.com/mrkshared/mmanual/section11/chapter131/131b.jsp
www.nlm.nih.gov/medlineplus/druginfo/medmaster/a682277.html
www.rxlist.com/cgi/generic/heparin.htm

ADVANCED PRACTICES CHAPTER REFERENCES

www.afadvisor.org/blood_tests.asp
www.drugs.com/PDR/Persantine_Tablets.html-60k
www.healthsquare.com/newrx/per1331.htm
www.rxlist.com/cgi/generic2/dipyrid.htm

10 Ophthalmic Agents

CHAPTER OBJECTIVES

After completing this chapter, you should be able to:
1. Describe the basic anatomy of the eye.
2. Define terminology related to ophthalmic medications.
3. State the purpose of each category of ophthalmic medications.
4. List examples of ophthalmic medications in each category.
5. Describe how ophthalmic agents are used in surgery.

CHAPTER OUTLINE

I. Anatomy Review
  A. Accessory Structures
     1. Eyebrows
     2. Eyelids
     3. Eyelashes
     4. Lacrimal System
  B. The Globe (Eyeball)
     1. Fibrous Layer
     2. Vascular Layer
     3. Nervous Layer
II. Topical Ophthalmic Medication Administration
III. Categories of Ophthalmic Agents
  A. Enzymes
     1. Increase Rate and Extent of Nerve Block
     2. Break Down Zonula
  B. Irrigation Solutions
     1. Cleanse the Operative Site
     2. Keep the Cornea Moist
  C. Viscoelastic Agents/OVD
     1. Keep Anterior Chamber Expanded
     2. Prevent Injury to Surrounding Tissues
  D. Miotics
     1. Constrict the Pupil
     2. Reduce Intraocular Pressure
  E. Mydriatics and Cycloplegics
     1. Dilate the Pupil
     2. Paralyze Sphincter Muscle of the Iris
  F. Ointments and Lubricants
     1. Used to Apply Medications as Antibiotics
     2. Lubricate and Protect the Cornea
  G. Anesthetics
     1. Numb and Paralyze Eye Structures
     2. Local
     3. Regional Block
        a. Retrobulbar
        b. Peribulbar
  H. Antiglaucoma Agents
     1. Decrease Intraocular Pressure
     2. Categories of Medications Used
        a. Miotics
        b. Diuretics
        c. Beta-Adrenergic Blockers

71

I. Anti-inflammatory Agents
1. Steroids
2. Nonsteroidal Anti-inflammatory Drugs (NSAIDs)
J. Diagnostic Agents
IV. Advanced Practices for the Surgical First Assistant

CHAPTER CONTENT MASTERY

Learning the Language (Key Terms)

Using your textbook or a standard medical dictionary, look up and write the definition of each term.

1. Constrict: _____

2. Cycloplegic: _____

3. Dilate: _____

4. Glaucoma: _____

5. Miotic: _____

6. Mydriatic: _____

7. NSAIDs: _____

8. OVD: _____

9. Proteolytic: _____

Chapter Review Questions

1. How are enzymes used in ophthalmic procedures?_____

_____

2. In which ophthalmic procedures would irrigation solutions be used?_____

_____

3. What is OVD? Why is this term used rather than viscoelastic agent?_____

_____

4. Why would lubricants be used in ophthalmic procedures?_____

_____

5. What is the difference between a miotic and a mydriatic agent?_____

_____

6. How can using lubricants result in corneal damage?_____

_____

7. What is the difference between a retrobulbar and a peribulbar block?_____

_____

8. Name two agents commonly used for local ophthalmic anesthesia._____

_____

9. How does each of the antiglaucoma medications mentioned work?_____

_____

10. List the steps for proper administration of topical ophthalmic medications. _____

_____

_____

Critical Thinking

1. Obtain a list of ophthalmic medications used at your facility and answer the following questions.
   a. What local anesthetic medications are used?
   b. What viscoelastic agents are used?
   c. What miotics are used?
   d. What mydriatics and cycloplegics are used?
2. Do anesthesia personnel at your facility use ointments to help protect patients' eyes? If yes, what

   ointments are used?_____

_____

3. List two ways in which aseptic technique is used to help prevent infections during ophthalmic surgery.

_____

_____

_____

_____

73

Identify the anatomic eye structures (Fig. 10–1 in the textbook) by labeling the drawing.

Word list: anterior chamber, central artery and vein, choroid, ciliary body, conjunctiva, cornea, fovea, iris, lateral rectus muscle, lens, limbus, medial rectus muscle, optic disk, optic nerve, posterior cavity, posterior chamber, pupil, retinal arteries and veins, retina, sclera, suspensory ligaments, visual axis

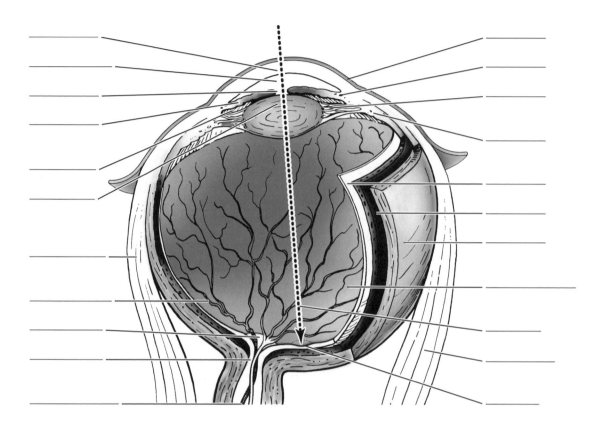

Utilizing Pharmacology Resources

1. Look up Miotics and Mydriatics in *Mosby's Drug Consult.* Answer the following questions:

   a. What medications are listed under each?_____

   _____

   _____

   b. What are the indications for usage of each?_____

   _____

   _____

   c. What are the contraindications for each?_____

   _____

   _____

2. Select one pharmacology source and complete a medication information worksheet for Timoptic. (Note: There are special references for ophthalmic medications.)

Internet Exercises

Go to www.glaucoma.com and answer the following questions:

1. What foundation is listed at this site? _____

_____

2. What is its goal? _____

_____

_____

3. List five important facts you learned at this site. _____

_____

_____

_____

_____

_____

1. The _____ is called the "window" of the eye.

2. A blockage of the trabecular meshwork that results in increased intraocular pressure results in a condition called _____.

3. The most common ophthalmic irrigating solution is _____.
4. Irrigation solutions do all of the following EXCEPT
   A. Moisten the cornea
   B. Decrease intraocular pressure
   C. Remove blood from the operative site
   D. Flush debris from the operative site

5. _____ are medications that constrict the pupil.

6. _____ are paralytic agents used to dilate the pupil.
7. In what type of block are the medications injected near the optic nerve?
   A. Spinal
   B. Retrobulbar
   C. Peribulbar
   D. Epidural

8. The acronym NSAIDs stands for _____.
9. Steroids are used in ophthalmics to
   A. Treat infection
   B. Dilate the pupils
   C. Decrease corneal inflammation
   D. Irrigate the cornea
10. How are ophthalmic dyes instilled?
    A. Intravenously
    B. Topically
    C. Regionally
    D. Intrathecally

ADVANCED PRACTICES CONTENT MASTERY

Learning the Language (Key Terms)
Using your textbook or a standard medical dictionary, look up and write the definition of each term.

1. Extracapsular: _____

2. Intracapsular: _____

3. Phacoemulsification: _____

Advanced Practices Chapter Review Questions
1. Eye medications are considered
   A. Potent
   B. Weak
   C. Short acting
   D. Long acting
2. Multiple dosages of mydriatic drops may be needed to achieve pupil dilation on a patient with
   A. Blue eyes
   B. Brown eyes
   C. Glaucoma
   D. Diabetes

3. Which of the following agents would be used to achieve maximum pupil dilation?
   A. Neo-Synephrine
   B. Miostat
   C. Carbachol
   D. Timoptic
4. Betamethasone is what type of pharmacologic agent?
   A. Anti-inflammatory
   B. Antibiotic
   C. Diuretic
   D. Vasoconstrictor
5. Substances used to lubricate and support the shape of the eye during lens extraction include all of the following EXCEPT
   A. Healon
   B. Provisc
   C. Viscoat
   D. Miochol
6. The ophthalmic condition commonly treated with a miotic drug is
   A. Cataract
   B. Retinal detachment
   C. Pterygium
   D. Glaucoma

CHAPTER REFERENCES

Gutierrez K: Pharmacotherapeutics: Clinical Decision-Making in Nursing. Philadelphia, WB Saunders, 1999.
Hopper T: Mosby's Pharmacy Technician: Principles and Practice. Philadelphia, WB Saunders, 2004.
Kee JL, Hayes ER: Pharmacology: A Nursing Process Approach, 3rd ed. Philadelphia, WB Saunders, 2000.
Martini FH: Fundamentals of Anatomy and Physiology, 5th ed. Upper Saddle River, NJ, Prentice Hall, 2001.
Netter FH: Atlas of Human Anatomy, 2nd ed. Teterboro, NJ, Novarlis, 1997.
O'Toole M: Miller-Keane Encyclopedia & Dictionary of Medicine, Nursing, and Allied Health, 7th ed. Philadelphia, WB Saunders, 2005.
Phillips N: Berry and Kohn's Operating Room Technique, 10th ed. St Louis, Mosby, 2004.
Rothrock JC: Alexander's Care of the Patient in Surgery, 12th ed. St Louis, Mosby, 2003.
www.aao.org/aao/education/library/memberalert/wydase1.cfm
www.alconlabs.com/ca_en/aj/products/duovisc-hpj.html
www.ashp.org/shortage/hyaluronidase.cfm
www.bausch.com/us/resource/surgical/cataract/viscoelastics.jsp
www.drugs.com/PDR/IC_Green.html
www.drugs.com/PDR/miochol_E_system_pak.html
www.drugs.com/PDR/ocucoat.html
www.escrs.org/journal/September2002/editsep02.asp
www.eyes.org/common/attachments/articles/diagnostic_dyes.pdf
www.healthdigest.org/drugs/pilocarpinehydrochloride.html
www.istavision.com/products/vitrase_package_insert.pdf
www.rxlist.com/egi/generic3/provisc.htm
www.rxmed.com

ADVANCED PRACTICES CHAPTER REFERENCES

Gutierrez K: Pharmacotherapeutics: Clinical Decision-Making in Nursing. Philadelphia, WB Saunders, 1999.
Lewis SM, Heitkemper MM, Dirksen SR: Medical Surgical Nursing: Assessment and Management of Clinical Problems, 5th ed. St Louis, Mosby, 2000.
Rothrock JC: Alexander's Care of the Patient in Surgery, 12th ed. St Louis, Mosby, 2003.
www.emedicine.com/oph/topic49.htm
www.merckfrosst.ca/e/products/timoptic/home.html
www.rxlist.com/cgi/generic/oflox.htm

11 Fluids and Irrigation Solutions

After completing this chapter, you should be able to:
1. Briefly describe the physiology of fluid loss in the surgical patient.
2. List fluid electrolytes and their functions crucial to homeostasis.
3. Define terms and abbreviations related to fluid replacement.
4. State objectives of parenteral fluid therapy in surgery.
5. List common intravenous solutions and their purposes in surgery.
6. List supplies needed to start an intravenous line.
7. List basic functions and types of blood.
8. State average adult circulating volume of blood, hemoglobin, and hematocrit values.
9. List the formed elements present in blood.
10. Define terms and abbreviations related to blood.
11. Briefly describe antigen–antibody interactions in blood types.
12. List and describe indications for blood replacement in the surgical patient.
13. List available options for blood replacement.
14. Describe components of whole blood used for replacement.
15. Define autologous and homologous blood donation.
16. Describe the process of intraoperative autotransfusion.
17. List volume expander solutions used in surgery.
18. List blood substitutes used in clinical trials.
19. Describe the procedure for blood replacement in surgery using donor blood from the blood bank.
20. List and describe fluids used as irrigation solutions in surgery.
21. List and describe supplies and equipment used for irrigation.

CHAPTER OUTLINE

I. Fluid and Electrolyte Management
  A. Physiology Review
  B. Intravenous Fluids
    1. Common Intravenous Fluids Administered in Surgery
      a. Sodium Chloride
        (1) Normal Saline 0.9%
        (2) $^1/_2$ Normal Saline 0.45%
        (3) $^1/_3$ Normal Saline 0.33%
        (4) $^1/_4$ Normal Saline 0.225%
      b. Dextrose
      c. Ionosol
      d. Normosol
      e. Lactated Ringer's (Hartmann's Solution)
      f. Plasma-lyte
      g. Isolyte E
    2. Intravenous Equipment and Supplies
      a. Angiocath
      b. Primary IV Tubing
      c. Secondary IV Tubing
II. Blood Replacement
  A. Physiology Review
    1. Functions of Blood
    2. Components of Blood
    3. Blood Typing
  B. Indications for Blood Replacement

79

C. Options for Blood Replacement
    1. Homologous Donation
        a. Whole Blood
        b. Packed Cells (RBCs)
        c. Plasma
        d. Platelets
        e. Cryoprecipitate
    2. Autologous Donation
        a. Self-donation
        b. Autotransfusion
    3. Volume Expanders
        a. Albumin
        b. Plasma Protein Fraction
        c. Dextran
        d. Hetastarch
    4. Blood Substitutes
        a. Hemopure
        b. PolyHeme
        c. Oxyglobin
D. Procedure for Donor Blood Replacement in Surgery
III. Irrigation Solutions
  A. Basic Irrigation Solutions
    1. Sodium Chloride
    2. Sterile Water
    3. PhysioSol
  B. Irrigation Solutions Used in Specialty Procedures
    1. 3% Sorbitol
    2. 1.5% Glycine
    3. Hyskon
  C. Synovial Fluid Replacement
  D. Irrigation Equipment and Supplies
    1. Bulb Syringe
    2. Asepto Syringe
    3. Standard Syringe
    4. Continuous Irrigation Systems
    5. Endoscopic Irrigation Systems
IV. Advanced Practices for the Surgical First Assistant

CHAPTER CONTENT MASTERY

Learning the Language (Key Terms)

Using your textbook or a standard medical dictionary, look up and write the definition of each term.

1. Antibody: _____

2. Antigen: _____

3. Arrhythmia: _____

4. Autologous: _____

5. Autotransfusion: _____

6. Electrolyte: _____

7. Hematocrit: _____

8. Hemoglobin: _____

9. Hemolysis: _____

10. Homologous: _____

11. Hypercalcemia: _____

12. Hyperkalemia: _____

13. Hypernatremia: _____

14. Hypocalcemia: _____

15. Hypokalemia: _____

16. Hyponatremia: _____

17. Hypovolemia: _____

18. Intravenous: _____

19. Isotonic: _____

20. Metabolic acidosis: _____

Chapter Review Questions

1. What are the basic functions of blood?_____

   _____

2. What is the average circulating blood volume in an adult?_____

   _____

3. Which surgical patients may require blood replacement?_____

   _____

4. What are the formed elements of blood? What is the main purpose of each?_____

   _____

   _____

   _____

5. What is hemoglobin? Hematocrit? What are the normal ranges in adults?_____

   _____

   _____

6. What are two electrolytes that have particular importance to the surgical patient? Why?_____

   _____

7. What common IV fluids are used in surgery? What is the purpose of each?_____

   _____

   _____

8. List two reasons to "start" an IV on the surgical patient preoperatively._____

   _____

   _____

9. What is the primary reason for the surgical patient to received blood replacement?_____

   _____

   _____

10. What is the difference between homologous and autologous donation?_____

   _____

   _____

Critical Thinking

1. Sodium chloride 0.9% is said to be isotonic. Why is this the irrigation solution of choice for most

   surgical procedures?_____

   _____

   _____

2. What should be considered when giving a dextrose IV solution to a diabetic patient?

_____

_____

3. What are some of the risks involved when giving the patient a transfusion of whole blood?

_____

_____

4. What should the surgical technologist consider and be prepared for when the surgical patient is given

large amounts of donor blood?_____

_____

_____

Scenario

You are assigned to the GU room for the day. The first procedure is a TURP on a 55-year-old man with an enlarged prostate gland.

1. What type of irrigation solution will be used?_____

_____

2. Why is this solution used on this procedure?_____

_____

3. Why must the rate of flow and the total volume of the solution used be carefully monitored?

_____

_____

Internet Exercises

Do an Internet search to find articles on the latest research concerning artificial blood products. Why is this research so important? What is being done at this time to develop new products? What are the disadvantages to artificial blood?

_____

_____

_____

_____

_____

_____

_____

_____

_____

_____

1. Sodium chloride IV solution is used when transfusing blood because it
   A. Adds calories to blood cells
   B. Warms the blood
   C. Does not hemolyze blood cells
   D. Does not conduct heat

2. Normal potassium levels for an adult are _____ mEq/L.

3. Too much calcium in the body is known as _____.

4. Another name for 0.9% sodium chloride is _____.

5. Another name for Hartmann's solution is _____ and it is a physiologic salt solution used

   to _____.

6. The four major groupings of blood types are_____.

7. Plasma may be administered when _____ is/are needed.
   A. Clotting factors
   B. Circulating volume
   C. RBCs
   D. Calories

8. An example of a volume expander is_____.
9. An irrigation solution that is used on a TURP and hysteroscopy is
   A. Sterile water
   B. Normal saline
   C. PhysioSol
   D. Glycine
10. Irrigating syringes include all of the following EXCEPT
    A. Asepto
    B. Insulin
    C. Bulb
    D. Regular

ADVANCED PRACTICES CONTENT MASTERY

Learning the Language (Key Terms)

Using your textbook or a standard medical dictionary, look up and write the definition of each term.

1. Hypertonic: _____

2. Hypotonic: _____

3. Osmolarity: _____

4. Osmosis: _____

5. Solute: _____

6. Solution: _____

7. Solvent: _____

ADVANCED PRACTICES CHAPTER REVIEW QUESTIONS

1. Why is normal saline considered an isotonic solution?_____

   _____

   _____

2. Which type of solution will make the cell shrink? Why?_____

   _____

3. What is the difference between continuous and intermittent IV administrations? Give examples of

   each._____

   _____

CHAPTER REFERENCES

Gutierrez K: Pharmacotherapeutics: Clinical Decision-Making in Nursing. Philadelphia, WB Saunders, 1999.
Kee JL, Hayes ER: Pharmacology: A Nursing Process Approach, 3rd ed. Philadelphia, WB Saunders, 2000.
Martini F: Fundamentals of Anatomy and Physiology, 5th ed. Upper Saddle River, NJ, Prentice Hall, 2001.
O'Toole M: Miller-Keane Encyclopedia & Dictionary of Medicine, Nursing, and Allied Health, 7th ed. Philadelphia, WB Saunders, 2005.
Phillips N: Berry and Kohn's Operating Room Technique, 10th ed. St Louis, Mosby, 2004.
Pickar GD: Dosage Calculations, 6th ed. Albany, Delmar, 1999.
Price P (exec. ed.): AST: Surgical Technology for the Surgical Technologist, 2nd ed. Clifton Park, NY, Thomson/Delmar Learning, 2004.
Rothrock JC: Alexander's Care of the Patient in Surgery, 12th ed. St Louis, Mosby, 2003.
ashp.org/shortage/drug.cfm
www.abbott.com
www.baxter.com
www.braun.com
www.drugs.com/meds/rhogam
www.emedicine.com/emerg/topic263.htm
www.ncbi.nlm.nih.gov/entrez/query.fcgi?cmd=Retrieve&db=PubMed&list_uids=14
www.shoulderdoc.co.uk/patient_info/viscoseal.asp

ADVANCED PRACTICES CHAPTER REFERENCES

Gutierrez K: Pharmacotherapeutics: Clinical Decision-Making in Nursing. Philadelphia, WB Saunders, 1999.
Josephson DL: Intravenous Infusion Therapy for Nurses: Principles and Practice. Albany, Delmar, 1999.
Kee JL, Hayes ER: Pharmacology: A Nursing Process Approach, 3rd ed. Philadelphia, WB Saunders, 2000.
Martini F: Fundamentals of Anatomy and Physiology, 5th ed. Upper Saddle River, NJ, Prentice Hall, 2001.
O'Toole M (ed): Miller-Keane Encyclopedia & Dictionary of Medicine, Nursing & Allied Health, 7th ed. Philadelphia, WB Saunders, 2005.

12 Antineoplastic Chemotherapy Agents

CHAPTER OBJECTIVES

After completing this chapter, you should be able to:
1. Define terms related to cancer.
2. Discuss different types of abnormal cell growth.
3. List the classifications of antineoplastic agents.
4. Define biologic response modifiers.
5. List the most prevalent carcinogen in the United States.
6. Discuss nanotechnology and its applications in medicine.

CHAPTER OUTLINE

I. Cancer Terminology
   A. Carcinoma
   B. CA
   C. Neoplasm
      1. Benign
      2. Malignant
II. Chemotherapy Agents
   A. Terminology
      1. Antineoplastic
      2. Cytotoxic
      3. Remission
   B. Alkylating Medications
   C. Antimetabolites
   D. Mitotic Inhibitors
   E. Antineoplastic Antibiotics
   F. Hormones and Hormone Antagonists
III. Biologic Response Modifiers
IV. Study of Disease
   A. Epidemiology
   B. Etiology
   C. Carcinogens
V. Antineoplastics for the Future
   A. Angiogenesis Inhibitors
   B. Nanotechnology

CHAPTER CONTENT MASTERY

Learning the Language (Key Terms)

Using your textbook or a standard medical dictionary, look up and write the definition of each term.

1. Antineoplastic: _____

2. Benign: _____

3. Cancer: _____

4. Carcinogen: _____

5. Cytotoxic: _____

6. Epidemiology: _____

7. Etiology: _____

8. Malignant: _____

9. Metastasis: _____

10. Neoplasm: _____

11. Remission: _____

Chapter Review Questions

1. What occurs in cells before cancer can start?_____

   _____

2. Describe the difference in the cell makeup of benign and malignant tumors._____

   _____

   _____

3. Why is an established schedule for dosage of chemotherapy agents important?_____

   _____

   _____

4. What is the largest group of anticancer agents?_____

   _____

5. Describe how each of the following chemotherapy medications works.

   a. Alkylating medications_____

   _____

   b. Antimetabolites_____

   _____

   c. Mitotic inhibitors_____

   _____

   d. Antineoplastic antibiotics_____

   _____

   e. Hormones and hormone antagonists_____

   _____

   f. Angiogenesis inhibitors_____

   _____

6. What is the purpose of BRMs?_____

   _____

7. Give two examples of BRM agents._____

   _____

8. Give an example of a carcinogen._____

9. List three possible uses for nanotechnology._____

   _____

   _____

89

Critical Thinking

1. Why would a chest radiograph be performed preoperatively on a patient with head and neck

cancer?_____

_____

_____

2. When would you have a patient come to surgery who is receiving chemotherapy? Give examples.

_____

_____

_____

Utilizing Pharmacology Resources

Look up Antineoplastics, Antibiotics in *Mosby's Drug Consult*. Select one of the medications listed and give the following information:

1. Name_____

2. Indications and usage_____

_____

_____

_____

3. Contraindications_____

_____

_____

4. Adverse reactions_____

_____

_____

5. Is this medication used for cure of disease or as a palliative measure?_____

_____

Internet Exercises

1. Search the Internet for current research on nanotechnology. What are the latest applications for this

technology in medicine?_____

_____

_____

_____

2. Search the Internet for the latest developments in chemotherapy agents. Choose a new agent and prepare a short report giving the agent's name, uses, side effects, and when it is expected to be given market approval.
3. Go to www.nci.nih.gov and select from: Cancer Topics, Clinical Trials, or Cancer Statistics. Prepare a brief presentation using information from one of these topics.

90

1. Another name for a tumor is _____.
2. If a tumor is benign, this means its cells
    A. Multiply rapidly
    B. Are unorganized
    C. Can invade surrounding tissues
    D. Are highly organized
3. Cytotoxic is defined as
    A. Destructive to cells
    B. Invasive to surrounding tissues
    C. Disruptive to the circulatory system
    D. Resembling normal body functions

4. The abatement or stopping of symptoms and possible cure of the disease is called _____.

5. The relief of symptoms without cure is termed _____.
6. The first antineoplastic drug(s) was/were
    a. 5 fluorouracil
    b. Nitrogen mustard
    c. Methotrexate
    d. Hormones
7. The antineoplastic drug used for ectopic pregnancy is
    a. Methotrexate
    b. 5-FU
    c. Bleomycin sulfate
    d. Tamoxifen
8. Hormones (corticosteroids) are used in antineoplastic therapy to act as
    a. Antibiotics
    b. Tumor cell inhibitors
    c. Enzyme inhibitors
    d. Anti-inflammatory agents
9. Interferons and interleukins work by all of the following EXCEPT
    a. Destroying white blood cells
    b. Boosting the immune system
    c. Interfering with tumor activity
    d. Promoting differentiation of stem cells

10. The term for "the cause of a disease" is _____.

CHAPTER REFERENCES

Gutierrez K: Pharmacotherapeutics: Clinical Decision-Making in Nursing. Philadelphia, WB Saunders, 1999.
Kee JL, Hayes ER: Pharmacology: A Nursing Process Approach, 3rd ed. Philadelphia, WB Saunders, 2000.
Hopper T: Mosby's Pharmacy Technician: Principles and Practice. Philadelphia, WB Saunders, 2004.
O'Toole M (ed): Miller-Keane Encyclopedia & Dictionary of Medicine, Nursing, and Allied Health, 7th ed. Philadelphia, WB Saunders, 2005.
nano.cancer.gov/nanotech_ncl.asp
www.babycenter.com
www.mc.vanderbilt.edu/reporter/?ID=2666

13 Preoperative Medications

CHAPTER OBJECTIVES

After completing this chapter, you should be able to:
1. Define terminology related to preoperative medications.
2. Identify the purpose of preoperative patient evaluation.
3. List sources of patient information used for preoperative evaluation.
4. List the components of a preoperative evaluation.
5. Identify classification of preoperative medications.
6. Identify the purpose of each group of preoperative medications.
7. State examples of medications in each classification.

CHAPTER OUTLINE

I. Preoperative Evaluation
   A. Purpose
   B. Sources of Data
   C. Assessment of Medical Conditions
   D. Components of Evaluation
   E. Physical Status Classification
II. Preoperative Medications
   A. Sedatives
   B. Analgesics
   C. Anticholinergics
   D. Gastric Agents
III. Advanced Practices for the Surgical First Assistant

CHAPTER CONTENT MASTERY

Learning the Language (Key Terms)
Using your textbook or a standard medical dictionary, look up and write the definition of each term.

1. Amnestic: _____

2. Analgesia: _____

3. Anesthesiologist: _____

4. Anterograde: _____

5. Anticholinergic: _____

6. Antisialagogue: _____

7. Anxiolysis: _____

8. Aspiration: _____

9. Benzodiazepine: _____

10. CRNA: _____

93

11. Hematocrit: _____

12. Hemoglobin: _____

13. Mcg/kg: _____

14. Mg/kg: _____

15. NPO: _____

16. Opioid: _____

17. Sedative: _____

18. Vagolysis: _____

Chapter Review Questions

1. Why is a preoperative evaluation conducted?

_____

2. What are the four categories of preoperative medications?

_____

_____

3. What is the purpose of each of the following types of drugs?
   (a) sedatives (b) opioids (c) anticholinergics (d) antacids (e) antiemetics (f) H2 blockers

   (a) _____ (b) _____ (c) _____

   (d) _____ (e) _____ (f) _____

4. State an example of a drug in each of the categories listed in question 3.

   _____ , _____ , _____ ,

   _____ , _____ , _____

Critical Thinking

Scenario

Mr. O'Neill is a very nervous, obese 61-year-old man with a history of diabetes and GERD. He is scheduled for an open reduction and internal fixation of a distal tibial fracture. He received a preoperative dose of 2 mg of midazolam (Versed) 15 minutes before being brought into the operating room. As he is settled on the operating room bed, the circulator begins to explain the importance of postoperative wound care to Mr. O'Neill.

1. In addition to midazolam, which other categories of preoperative medications do you think Mr. O'Neill

   will have received and why? _____

   _____

2. Is this the appropriate time to instruct Mr. O'Neill regarding his wound care? Why or why not?

   _____

Visual Exercises

Complete a preanesthesia questionnaire, located at the end of this chapter, as if you were the patient. Now, review the questionnaire as if you were the anesthesia provider. What risk factors do you notice? What preoperative medications would you order?

_____

_____

Utilizing Pharmacology Resources

1. Complete a medication information sheet on midazolam (Versed) using two different resources.

   a. Which source did you find most helpful and why? _____

   b. Which information was the most difficult to find? _____

Internet Exercises

1. Using a favorite search engine, look up the drug glycopyrrolate (Robinul).

   a. How many "hits" did you get? _____

   b. List two of the websites the search engine found for you.

   _____

   _____

   c. Visit one of the websites you think is most reliable.

   d. What was the most helpful information found on that site? _____

   e. How will the information you learned help you in clinical practice? _____

   _____

2. Using the same search engine, look up metoclopramide (Reglan).

   a. How many "hits" did you get? _____

   b. List two different websites the search engine found for you. Do not use sites you used in the previous exercise.

   _____

   _____

   c. Visit one of the websites you think is most reliable.

   d. What was the most helpful information found on that site? _____

   _____

CHAPTER QUIZ

1. Define the term *anterograde*.

_____

2. What does the abbreviation mg/kg mean? _____
3. List two sources of patient information used for preoperative evaluation.

_____ and _____
4. Match the following categories of preoperative medications with their purpose.

_____ analgesic   a. anxiolysis

_____ anticholinergic   b. dry secretions

_____ gastric agent   c. prevent reflux

_____ sedative   d. reduce pain

5. Which of the following is an analgesic?
   A. Atropine (Atropine)
   B. Meperidine (Demerol)
   C. Midazolam (Versed)
   D. Ondansetron (Zofran)
6. Glycopyrrolate (Robinul) is a/an
   A. Analgesic
   B. Anticholinergic
   C. Gastric agent
   D. Sedative

ADVANCED PRACTICES CONTENT MASTERY

Learning the Language (Key Terms)

Using your textbook or a standard medical dictionary, look up and write the definition of each term.
1. Bowel prep:

_____

2. Convulsions:

_____

3. Hypertension:

_____

Advanced Practices Chapter Review Questions

1. Which procedures will require a preoperative bowel prep? Why? _____

_____

2. How is the resident bacteria found in the bowel eliminated? _____

3. How do anticonvulsants work? _____

4. Name the groups of medications used to treat hypertension. _____

_____

CHAPTER REFERENCES

Duke J: Anesthesia Secrets, 2nd ed. Philadelphia, Hanley and Belfus, 2000.
Nagelhout J, Zaglaniczny K, Haglund V: Handbook of Nurse Anesthesia, 2nd ed. Philadelphia, WB Saunders, 2001.
Saeb-Parsy K, Assomull RG, Khan FZ, et al: Instant Pharmacology. Chichester, England, Wiley and Sons, 1999.
Simpson P, Popat M: Understanding Anesthesia, 4th ed. Edinburgh, Butterworth Heineman, 2000.
www.aana.com/
www.aana.com/patients/preop.asp
www.asahq.org/
www.fpnotebook.com/SUR42.htm
www.medvarsity.com/vmu1.2/dmr/dmrdata/drug/Preoperative%20Medication.htm
www.quia.com/mc/337608.html
www.tsa.org/public_resources/ambulatory_surgery.html
www.uhcanesthesia.com/PAT/Surgeons/pat-surg-info/view

ADVANCED PRACTICES CHAPTER REFERENCES

Cameron JL: Current Surgical Therapy. St Louis, Mosby, 2001.
Gutierrez K: Pharmacotherapeutics: Clinical Decision-Making in Nursing. Philadelphia, WB Saunders, 1999.
Kaplan NM, Ram CVS: Individualized therapy of hypertension. N Engl J Med 333:396, 1995.
Kee JL, Hayes ER: Pharmacology: A Nursing Process Approach. Philadelphia, WB Saunders, 2003.
Khatri V, Asensio JA: Operative Surgery Manual. Philadelphia, WB Saunders, 2003.
www.healthsquare.com/hbp5.htm

Chapter **13** **Preoperative Medications**

Preanesthesia Questionnaire

The information you supply below assists in the development of your anesthesia care.
Please complete this questionnaire accurately and completely.

Patient Name _____

Age _____ Weight _____ Height _____ Date _____

Allergies _____

_____

Current Medications (Prescription and Nonprescription)_____

_____

Prior Operations _____

_____

Preanesthesia Questionnaire

Please answer the following questions. These responses will help us provide the anesthetic that is best for you.

Yes	No	Question
[ ]	[ ]	Have you recently had a cold or the flu?
[ ]	[ ]	Are you allergic to latex (rubber) products?
[ ]	[ ]	Have you experienced chest pain?
[ ]	[ ]	Do you have a heart condition?
[ ]	[ ]	Do you have hypertension (high blood pressure)?
[ ]	[ ]	Do you experience shortness of breath?
[ ]	[ ]	Do you have asthma, bronchitis, or any other breathing problem?
[ ]	[ ]	Do you (or did you) smoke?
		Packs/day _____. Number of years _____.
		Date you quit _____.
[ ]	[ ]	Do you consume alcohol?
		Drinks/week _____.
[ ]	[ ]	Do you take or have you taken recreational drugs?
[ ]	[ ]	Have you taken cortisone (steroids) in the last six months?
[ ]	[ ]	Do you have diabetes?
[ ]	[ ]	Have you had hepatitis, liver disease, or jaundice?
[ ]	[ ]	Do you have a thyroid condition?
[ ]	[ ]	Do you have or have you had kidney disease?
[ ]	[ ]	Do you have ulcers or other stomach disorders?
[ ]	[ ]	Do you have a hiatal hernia?
[ ]	[ ]	Do you have back or neck pain?
[ ]	[ ]	Do you have numbness, weakness, or paralysis of your extremities?
[ ]	[ ]	Do you have any muscle or nerve disease?
[ ]	[ ]	Do you or any of your family have sickle cell trait?
[ ]	[ ]	Have you or any blood relatives had difficulties with anesthesia?
[ ]	[ ]	Do you have bleeding problems?
[ ]	[ ]	Do you have loose, chipped, false teeth, or bridgework?
[ ]	[ ]	Do you have any oral piercings, (such as studs or rings) in your tongue or lip?
[ ]	[ ]	Do you wear contact lenses?
[ ]	[ ]	Have you ever received a blood transfusion?
[ ]	[ ]	(Women) Are you pregnant?
		Due date _____.

From American Association of Nurse Anesthetists: AANA's Public Information and Patient Resources Center, 2005, www.aana.com/patients/preop.asp, accessed October 4, 2005.

14 Patient Monitoring and Local and Regional Anesthesia

CHAPTER OBJECTIVES

After completing this chapter, you should be able to:
1. Define terminology related to patient monitoring and anesthesia.
2. Describe types of patient-monitoring devices.
3. Compare and contrast local anesthesia, monitored anesthesia care, and regional anesthesia.
4. List surgical procedures that may be performed under local or regional anesthesia.
5. Identify common agents used in local anesthesia and regional anesthesia.
6. Discuss the use of epinephrine in local anesthetic agents.
7. Describe types of regional blocks.

CHAPTER OUTLINE

I. Patient Monitoring
   A. Electrocardiography
   B. Pulse Oximetry
   C. Blood Pressure
   D. Temperature
   E. Capnometry
   F. Monitoring Consciousness
   G. Neuromuscular Function
   H. Advanced Monitoring
II. Local and Regional Anesthesia
   A. Local Anesthesia
      1. Applications for Local Anesthesia
      2. Agents Used for Local Anesthesia
      3. Monitored Anesthesia Care
   B. Regional Anesthesia
      1. Spinal Anesthesia
      2. Epidural Anesthesia
      3. Caudal Block
      4. Retrobulbar Block
      5. Extremity Block
III. Advanced Practices for the Surgical First Assistant

CHAPTER CONTENT MASTERY

Learning the Language (Key Terms)

Using your textbook or a standard medical dictionary, look up and write the definition of each term.

1. ABGs: _____

2. Asystole: _____

3. Auscultation: _____

4. Blood pressure: _____

5. Bradycardia: _____

6. Capnometry: _____

7. CVP line: _____

8. Dysrhythmias: _____

9. Electrocardiography: _____

10. Electroencephalogram: _____

11. Epidural: _____

12. Exsanguination: _____

13. Intrathecally: _____

14. Laryngospasm: _____

15. Local anesthesia: _____

16. Monitored anesthesia care (MAC): _____

17. Precordial: _____

18. Pulse oximetry: _____

19. PVC: _____

20. Regional anesthesia: _____

21. Tachycardia: _____

22. Vasoconstrictor: _____

23. Vasodilation: _____

Chapter Review Questions

1. Describe three different types of monitoring devices including definition, purpose, and equipment used. _____

_____

2. How does local anesthesia differ from monitored anesthesia care? How are the two methods alike?

_____

3. List three surgical procedures that may be performed under local anesthesia.

_____

4. What patient factors may indicate the need for monitored anesthesia care? _____

_____

5. Describe two types of regional anesthesia including definition, purpose, and method. _____

_____

Critical Thinking

Scenario 1

Ms. Ortiz is a 78-year-old woman with emphysema. She has recently undergone a hysterectomy for uterine cancer. The pelvic lymph nodes were positive for cancer. She has been admitted to surgery for placement of a venous access port for chemotherapy.

1. Would you select local anesthesia or monitored anesthesia care? Justify your answer.

_____

2. How would her medical condition affect the pulse oximetry measurements? Why?

_____

Scenario 2

Mr. Delano is a 69-year-old man admitted to surgery for placement of a transvenous pacemaker. The surgeon's preference card indicates that you should have 50 mL of 1% lidocaine with epinephrine 1:100,000 on the back table for injection.

1. Would you select local anesthesia or monitored anesthesia care? Justify your answer.

_____

2. Is the agent indicated on the preference card acceptable for this procedure? Why or why not?

_____

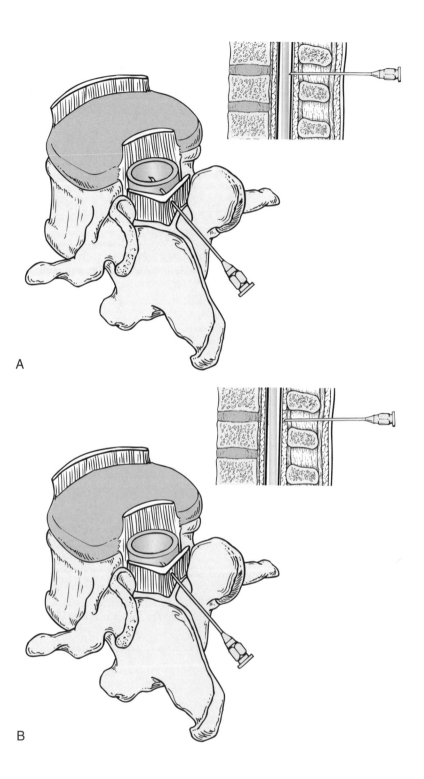

A

B

Identify which figure shows:

1. An epidural anesthesia location _____

2. A spinal anesthesia location _____

Utilizing Pharmacology Resources

1. Complete a medication information sheet on 1% lidocaine (Xylocaine) with epinephrine 1:100,000 using two different resources.

   a. Which source did you find most helpful and why? _____

   b. Which information was the most difficult to find? _____

2. Look up bupivacaine in a pharmacology resource other than your textbook.

   a. What strengths is it available in? _____

   b. What volumes? _____

   c. What are the contraindications for use? _____

Internet Exercises

1. Using a favorite search engine, look up capnometry.

   a. How many "hits" did you get? _____
   b. List two of the websites the search engine found for you.

   _____

   _____

   c. Visit one of the websites you think is most reliable.

   d. What was the most helpful information found on that site? _____

   _____

   e. How will the information you learned help you in clinical practice? _____

   _____

2. Using a different search engine, look up retrobulbar block.

   a. How many "hits" did you get? _____
   b. List two different websites the search engine found for you.

   _____

   _____

   c. Visit one of the websites you think is most reliable.

   d. What was the most helpful information found on that site? _____

   _____

       Chapter **14** **Patient Monitoring and Local and Regional Anesthesia**

1. Define the term *precordial*.

   _____

2. Capnometry means the measure of
   A. Tidal volume
   B. Oxygen saturation
   C. Expired carbon dioxide
   D. Vital capacity

3. Describe electrocardiography used as a monitoring device in surgery.

   _____

   _____

4. Which of the following monitoring devices is considered invasive?
   A. Pulse oximeter
   B. Sphygmomanometer
   C. Bispectral index monitor
   D. Arterial line

5. Which of the following types of anesthesia interrupts pain impulses at the nerve endings?
   A. Epidural anesthesia
   B. Extremity block
   C. Local anesthesia
   D. Caudal block

6. List two surgical applications for local anesthesia. _____

7. State an indication for monitored anesthesia care.

   _____

8. Which of the following local anesthetics is intended for topical use only?
   A. Cocaine
   B. Bupivacaine
   C. Lidocaine
   D. Mepivacaine

9. List a specific surgical procedure that may be performed under spinal anesthesia. _____

10. List a specific surgical procedure that may be performed under extremity block. _____

ADVANCED PRACTICES CONTENT MASTERY

Learning the Language (Key Terms)

Using your textbook or a standard medical dictionary, look up and write the definition of each term.

1. Circumoral: _____

2. Erythema: _____

3. PABA: _____

4. Urticaria: _____

Advanced Practices Chapter Review Questions

1. Explain the difference between aminoesters and aminoamides. _____

   _____

2. Why should patients with hepatitis be closely monitored while on amides? _____

   _____

3. Name the two principle adverse effects on the patient from local anesthetics. _____

_____

4. What is the difference between a local and a systemic allergic reaction? Give clinical signs of each.

_____

_____

5. What causes systemic toxicity of local anesthetics? Give two symptoms. _____

_____

6. Why can a larger volume of local anesthetics with epinephrine be injected into tissues without causing

    toxicity? _____

CHAPTER REFERENCES

Duke J: Anesthesia Secrets, 2nd ed. Philadelphia, Hanley and Belfus, 2000.
Nagelhout J, Zaglaniczny K, Haglund V: Handbook of Nurse Anesthesia, 2nd ed. Philadelphia, WB Saunders, 2001.
Saeb-Parsy K, Assomull RG, Khan FZ, et al: Instant Pharmacology. Chichester, England, Wiley and Sons, 1999.
Simpson P, Popat M: Understanding Anesthesia, 4th ed. Edinburgh, Butterworth Heineman, 2002.
anesthesiologyinfo.com/articles/12092002.php
www.aana.com/
www.ahcpr.gov/clinic/epcsums/anestsum.htm
www.asahq.org/
www.asanr.com/alternatives.html
www.drugs.com/PDR/Sensorcaine_MPF_Injection.html
www.drugs.com/PDR/Xylocaine_with_Epinephrine_Injection.html
www.emedicine.com/ent/topic20.htm
www.nlm.nih.gov/medlineplus/tutorials/epiduralanesthesia/htm/index.htm
www.nysora.com/techniques/axillary_brachial_plexus_block/
www.oximeter.org/pulseox/principles.htm

ADVANCED PRACTICES CHAPTER REFERENCES

Gutierrez K: Pharmacotherapeutics: Clinical Decision-Making in Nursing. Philadelphia, WB Saunders, 1999.
Kee JL, Hayes ER: Pharmacology: A Nursing Process Approach, 3rd ed. Philadelphia, WB Saunders, 2000.
Price P: AST, Surgical Technology for the Surgical Technologist, 2nd ed. Clifton Park, NY, Thomson Delmar Learning, 2004.
www.emedicine.com/emerg/topic761.htm
www.emedicine.com/orthoped/topic581.htm
www.virtual-anesthesia-textbook.com

15 General Anesthesia

CHAPTER OBJECTIVES

After completing this chapter, you should be able to:
1. Define terminology related to anesthesia.
2. Discuss indications for general anesthesia.
3. Identify anesthesia equipment.
4. Explain the basic components of a general anesthetic.
5. List methods of inducing general anesthesia.
6. Define the phases of general anesthesia.
7. Discuss options for airway management.
8. Describe the process of endotracheal intubation.
9. Discuss the concept of awareness under anesthesia.
10. List agents used to accomplish general anesthesia.
11. Identify the purposes and categories of agents used in general anesthesia.
12. Identify generic and trade names of common agents used in anesthesia.
13. State the phase of anesthesia in which various agents are administered.
14. Compare and contrast depolarizing and nondepolarizing muscle relaxants.

CHAPTER OUTLINE

I. Introduction to Anesthesia
   A. Patient Factors
   B. Desired Effects
   C. Equipment
II. Components of General Anesthesia
   A. Four Goals
   B. Administration Methods
III. Phases of General Anesthesia
   A. Preinduction Phase
   B. Induction Phase
      1. Airway Management
         a. Mask
         b. LMA
         c. Endotracheal tube
         d. Variation
   C. Maintenance Phase
      1. Awareness under Anesthesia
      2. Muscle Relaxation
   D. Emergence Phase
IV. Agents Used for General Anesthesia
   A. Intravenous Induction Agents
   B. Analgesics
   C. Inhalation Agents
   D. Neuromuscular Blocking Agents
      1. Muscle Physiology Review
      2. Muscle Relaxants
   E. Reversal Agents
V. Advanced Practices for the Surgical First Assistant

109

Learning the Language (Key Terms)

Using your textbook or a standard medical dictionary, look up and write the definition of each term.

1. Amnestic: _____

2. Anesthesia: _____

3. Depolarization: _____

4. Emergence phase: _____

5. Emulsion: _____

6. ET: _____

7. Extubation: _____

8. Fasciculation: _____

9. Induction phase: _____

10. Intubation: _____

11. Lacrimation: _____

12. LMA: _____

13. Maintenance phase: _____

14. Minimum alveolar concentration (MAC): _____

15. Nebulizer: _____

16. Opioid: _____

17. PACU: _____

18. Preinduction phase: _____

19. RSI: _____

20. Repolarization: _____

Chapter Review Questions

1. What are the four components of a general anesthetic? _____

_____

2. What two routes are used to deliver general anesthesia? _____

3. What is the scrubbed surgical technologist doing during each phase of a general anesthetic? What is

the circulating surgical technologist doing during each phase? _____

_____

4. Can you list common medications in each category of anesthetic agents? _____

5. Match generic and trade names of drugs used in anesthesia.

_____ desflurane		a. Anectine	
_____ fentanyl		b. Sublimaze	
_____ lidocaine		c. Suprane	
_____ succinylcholine		d. Xylocaine	

6. How do muscle relaxants work? _____

7. How are depolarizing and nondepolarizing muscle relaxants alike? How are they different?

_____

_____

Critical Thinking

Scenario 1

Mrs. Diaz is a 45-year-old woman. She sustained a fractured wrist when she slipped on an icy sidewalk exiting a restaurant. She has been admitted to surgery for closed reduction and cast application.

1. Which method of airway control do you think the anesthesia provider will select for Mrs. Diaz? Justify

your answer. _____

_____

Scenario 2

Johnny Duncan is a 5-year-old boy. He sustained a greenstick fracture of the forearm when he fell from a park swing set. He has been admitted to surgery for a closed reduction and cast application.

1. Which method of administration do you think the anesthesia provider will select for Johnny? Justify

your answer. _____

_____

Utilizing Pharmacology Resources

1. Complete a medication information sheet on propofol (Diprivan) using two different resources.

   a. Which source did you find most helpful and why? _____

   b. Which information was the most difficult to find? _____

2. Select an anesthesia textbook (for CRNAs or MDs) and look up intubation.

   a. How easy was the text to understand? _____

   b. How did the information help you understand the process of intubation? _____

_____

111

Internet Exercises

1. Visit the website for the American Association of Nurse Anesthetists (www.aana.org).

   a. What was the most helpful information found on that site? _____

   b. How will the information you learned help you in clinical practice? _____
   _____

2. Visit the website for the American Society of Anesthesiologists (www.asahq.org).

   a. What was the most helpful information found on that site? _____

   b. How will the information you learned help you in clinical practice? _____
   _____

   c. How did the site for anesthesiologists compare with the site for nurse anesthetists? _____
   _____

   d. Which site provided better information? _____

3. Using your favorite search engine, do a search for physiology of muscle contraction.

   a. How many "hits" did you get? _____
   b. Choose three that you think are reliable sites and explore them.
   c. Select the best of the three and bring a copy of the information to class for discussion.

1. Define the term *fasciculation*. _____
2. Which of the following conditions is an indication for general anesthesia?
   A. Cardiac dysfunction
   B. Cognitive impairment
   C. Short procedure duration
   D. Traumatic injury
3. Which of the following is NOT a basic component of a general anesthetic?
   A. Analgesia
   B. Dyskinesia
   C. Muscle relaxation
   D. Unconsciousness

4. The induction phase of general anesthesia begins with _____ and ends with

   _____ .

5. Which of the following options for airway management would most likely be indicated for a 68-year-old morbidly obese man with a short, thick neck admitted to surgery for ORIF of a cervical fracture?
   A. Awake intubation
   B. Laryngeal masked airway
   C. Masked airway
   D. Nasal intubation
6. Which of the following categories of agents are NOT used to accomplish general anesthesia?
   A. Barbiturates
   B. Cephalosporins
   C. Hypnotic agents
   D. Opioid analgesics
7. What is the purpose of a synthetic opioid?
   A. Amnesia
   B. Analgesia
   C. Muscle relaxation
   D. Unconsciousness
8. Which of the following agents used for general anesthesia is a potent analgesic?
   A. Etomidate (Amidate)
   B. Ketamine (Ketalar)
   C. Midazolam (Versed)
   D. Thiopental (Pentothal)
9. The generic name for Anectine is
   A. Naloxone
   B. Pancuronium
   C. Succinylcholine
   D. Tubocurarine
10. Which of the following agents may be administered in the emergence phase of general anesthesia?
    A. Methohexital (Brevital)
    B. Neostigmine (Prostigmin)
    C. Propofol (Diprivan)
    D. Vecuronium (Norcuron)

CHAPTER REFERENCES

Duke J: Anesthesia Secrets, 2nd ed. Philadelphia, Hanley and Belfus, 2000.
Nagelhout J, Zaglaniczny K, Haglund V: Handbook of Nurse Anesthesia, 2nd ed. Philadelphia, WB Saunders, 2001.
Saeb-Parsy K, Assomull RG, Khan FZ, et al: Instant Pharmacology. Chichester, England, Wiley and Sons, 1999.
Simpson P, Popat M: Understanding Anesthesia, 4th ed. Edinburgh, Butterworth Heinemann, 2002.
health.howstuffworks.com/anesthesia2.htm
vam.anest.ufl.edu/
www.aana.com/
www.amsa.org/surg/anescase2.cfm

www.asahq.org/
www.chclibrary.org/micromed/00037320.html
www.datex-ohmeda.com/clinical/cw_issue_07_article2.htm
www.emedicine.com/plastic/topic110.htm
www.nlm.nih.gov/medlineplus/tutorials/generalanesthesia/htm/index.htm
www.utmb.edu/otoref/Grnds/Anesthesia-200002/anesthesia-200002.htm

ADVANCED PRACTICES CHAPTER REFERENCES

O'Toole M (ed): Miller-Keane Encyclopedia & Dictionary of Medicine, Nursing, and Allied Health, 7th ed. Philadelphia, WB Saunders, 2005.
nccam.nih.gov/health/acupuncture/
www.cavalierdaily.com/CVArticle_print.asp?ID=19016&pid1132
www.holistic-online.com/acupuncture/acp_home.htm
www.medicalacupuncture.org
www.utmb.edu/otoref/grnds/chempeel.htm

16 Emergency Situations

CHAPTER OBJECTIVES

After completing this chapter, you should be able to:
1. Define terminology related to emergency situations.
2. Identify emergency situations associated with anesthesia.
3. Identify medications used in emergency situations.
4. State the purpose of drugs used in emergency situations.
5. Identify the category of specified emergency medications.
6. Discuss the role of the surgical technologist during a cardiac emergency in surgery.
7. List clinical signs of malignant hyperthermia.
8. Outline basic course of treatment for malignant hyperthermia.
9. Discuss the role of the surgical technologist in a malignant hyperthermia crisis.

CHAPTER OUTLINE

I. Respiratory Emergencies
   A. Bronchospasm
   B. Anaphylaxis
      1. Medication, Anesthetic, and Latex Reactions
      2. Transfusion (Hemolytic) Reaction
   C. Laryngospasm
II. Cardiac Arrest
   A. Causes
   B. Roles of the Operating Room Team
   C. Roles of the Surgical Technologist
      1. First scrub role
      2. Second assistant
      3. First/Surgical assistant
      4. Circulator
   D. Medications
   E. Miscellaneous Cardiovascular Drugs
      1. Adrenergic Agonists
      2. Adrenergic Antagonists
      3. Cholinergic Agents
      4. Antiarrhythmics
      5. Calcium Channel Blockers
      6. Vasodilators
      7. Inotropic Agents
III. Malignant Hyperthermia
   A. Clinical Signs of Malignant Hyperthermia
   B. Malignant Hyperthermia Treatment Protocol

CHAPTER CONTENT MASTERY

Learning the Language (Key Terms)

Using your textbook or a standard medical dictionary, look up and write the definition of each term.

1. Anaphylaxis: _____

2. Asystole: _____

3. Bolus: _____

4. Bradycardia: _____

5. Bronchospasm: _____

6. Capnography: _____

7. Cyanosis: _____

8. Desaturation: _____

9. Diaphoresis: _____

10. Hemoglobinuria: _____

11. Hypermetabolic: _____

12. Pyrexia: _____

13. Tachycardia: _____

14. Tachypnea: _____

15. Urticaria: _____

Chapter Review Questions

1. What are some anesthesia complications treated pharmacologically?

_____

2. What are the drugs used to treat those complications?

_____

3. Can you name some drugs used to treat cardiac arrest? What is the purpose of each?

_____

4. What are the signs of malignant hyperthermia?

_____

5. What are the basic treatment steps for MH?

_____

6. How would the circulating surgical technologist function during a cardiac emergency?

_____

Critical Thinking

Scenario 1

You have just finished first scrubbing for a tonsillectomy. While you are cleaning up, the patient is extubated and begins emitting a high-pitched "crowing" sound indicating that the patient is experiencing laryngospasm.

1. What steps do you take? _____

2. What steps does the anesthesia provider take? _____

Scenario 2

You are scheduled to scrub an abdominal aortic aneurysm repair on a 63-year-old man who has tested positive for malignant hyperthermia.

1. What additional preparations must be made for this patient and why? _____

_____

Scenario 3

It is 8 AM, and you have just scrubbed in to retract (second scrub role, not first scrub) on a gastric resection procedure. The patient is draped, but no incision has been made when anesthesia calls a code blue. The patient is in cardiac arrest.

1. Which basic duties will be performed by each team member? _____

_____

2. What duties might you be required to perform? _____

_____

Utilizing Pharmacology Resources

1. Complete a medication information sheet on dantrolene (Dantrium) using two different resources.

   a. Which source did you find most helpful and why? _____

   b. Which information was the most difficult to find? _____

2. Select two pharmacology resources (other than your textbook) and look up the medication dopamine (Intropin).

   a. In what medication category is dopamine? _____

   b. What is an indication for dopamine? _____

117

Internet Exercises

1. Using a favorite search engine, look up malignant hyperthermia.

   a. How many "hits" did you get? _____

   b. List two of the websites the search engine found for you.

      _____

      _____

   c. Visit one of the websites you think is most reliable.

   d. What was the most helpful information found on that site? _____

   e. How will the information you learned help you in clinical practice? _____

      _____

2. Go to the National Institutes of Health's website (www.nih.gov) and search the site for information on treatment for cardiac arrest.

   a. How many "hits" did you get? _____

   b. List three different types of references contained at the site. _____,

      _____, and _____

   c. Select one of the references, print it, highlight key points in the item, and bring it to class for discussion.

   d. What was the most helpful information found on that site? _____

      _____

CHAPTER QUIZ

1. Define the term *capnography*.

   _____

2. List two emergency situations associated with anesthesia.

   _____

   _____

3. Which of the following is NOT an antiarrhythmic agent?
   A. Amiodarone (Cordarone)
   B. Isoproterenol (Isuprel)
   C. Lidocaine (Xylocaine)
   D. Procainamide (Pronestyl)
4. The medication dobutamine (Dobutrex) may be used in the course of treatment for anaphylaxis to
   A. Decrease cardiac irritability
   B. Raise blood pressure
   C. Release antihistamines
   D. Treat bronchospasm
5. Which of the following medications is a beta-adrenergic agonist used in the treatment of bronchospasm?
   A. Albuterol (Proventil)
   B. Digoxin (Lanoxin)
   C. Nitroprusside (Nipride)
   D. Verapamil (Isoptin)
6. List two clinical signs of malignant hyperthermia. _____
7. Which of the following medications may most likely be administered during resuscitation for cardiac arrest?
   A. Amiodarone (Cordarone)
   B. Digoxin (Lanoxin)
   C. Labetalol (Normodyne)
   D. Vasopressin (Pitressin)
8. Which of the following categories of medications is used in the treatment of malignant hyperthermia?
   A. Antihypertensives
   B. Diuretics
   C. Inotropic agents
   D. Vasodilators

CHAPTER REFERENCES

Duke J: Anesthesia Secrets, 2nd ed. Philadelphia, Hanley and Belfus, 2000.
Nagelhout J, Zaglaniczny K, Haglund V: Handbook of Nurse Anesthesia, 2nd ed. Philadelphia, WB Saunders, 2001.
Saeb-Parsy K, Assomull RG, Khan FZ, et al: Instant Pharmacology. Chichester, England, Wiley and Sons, 1999.
Simpson P, Popat M: Understanding Anesthesia, 4th ed. Edinburgh, Butterworth Heineman, 2002.
www.aana.com/
www.acls.net/newalgo/vfpvt.htm
www.anes.ucla.edu/dept/mh.html
www.asahq.org/
www.medana.unibas.ch/eng/mh/mhtutori.htm
www.metrohealthanesthesia.com/edu/mh/mh_quiz.htm
www.mhaus.org/

Medication Information Worksheet

Medication (generic name and trade name):

_____

Specific source of medication information (e.g., reference book title, edition, and page number; or complete website address):

_____

Classification (and subcategory or subcategories):

_____

Source of drug:
   plant   animal   mineral   synthetic   semisynthetic   biotechnology
Drug form/s: solid   semisolid   liquid   gas
Drug dosage (adult):

_____

Indications for use (with emphasis on surgery):

_____

_____

Administration route or routes:

_____

List two side effects.

_____

List an adverse effect.

_____

What precautions are given?

_____

List drug interactions.

_____

What are the contraindications?

_____

What is the drug's action on two different body systems? (e.g., Does it depress respirations?)

_____

How is the drug absorbed?

_____

How is it distributed?

_____

How is the drug metabolized?

_____

How is the drug excreted?

_____

121

Anesthesia Worksheet

Name_____

Date_____

1. What is the name of your anesthesia provider?

2. What are his or her credentials (MD, DO, CRNA, other)?

3. What is the purpose of induction agents such as sodium pentothal, propofol, and etomidate?

4. Why do anesthesia personnel prepare propofol shortly before its use?

5. Which of the five senses is the last to leave and the first to return on the anesthetized patient?

6. Name three agents used for local and regional anesthetics.

7. Some local and regional anesthetics contain epinephrine, a vasoconstrictor. Why should they not be used to "block" digits?

8. What is a major risk factor in patient overdosage with local anesthetics?

9. Why is cocaine used as a topical anesthetic only?

10. Why do anesthesia personnel put eye lubricants in the patient's eyes before most surgical procedures?

11. Name one eye lubricant used at your site.

12. Where are the oral suction tips kept in your surgical room?

13. Why is it important for anesthesia personnel to have oral suction available, especially during extubation?

14. Why are special endotracheal tubes necessary for laser surgery for the oral area?

123

15. What is meant by "applying cricoid pressure" during intubation (especially during a rapid sequence induction)?

16. When should you release this cricoid pressure?

17. What is laryngospasm?

18. How is laryngospasm treated?

19. What does the pulse ox tell you?

20. Where is the pulse ox applied to the patient and how does it work?

21. What is the code for a cardiac arrest at your site?

22. Where is the equipment and protocol for malignant hyperthermia kept at your site?

23. Why do anesthesia personnel administer nitrous oxide with other gases during the operative procedure?

24. What is a jet ventilator?

25. List one piece of information you learned today.

Adverse reactions/side effects:

Contraindications:

Adverse reactions/side effects:

Contraindications:

Adverse reactions/side effects:

Contraindications:

Adverse reactions/side effects:

Contraindications:

Generic name: Classification:
                                       Schedule:

Brand names: Dosage forms:

Indications and usage: Dosage:

Generic name: Classification:
                                       Schedule:

Brand names: Dosage forms:

Indications and usage: Dosage:

Generic name: Classification:
                                       Schedule:

Brand names: Dosage forms:

Indications and usage: Dosage:

Generic name: Classification:
                                       Schedule:

Brand names: Dosage forms:

Indications and usage: Dosage:

Adverse reactions/side effects:

Contraindications:

Adverse reactions/side effects:

Contraindications:

Adverse reactions/side effects:

Contraindications:

Adverse reactions/side effects:

Contraindications:

Generic name: Classification:
                                        Schedule:

Brand names: Dosage forms:

Indications and usage:

                                        Dosage:

Generic name: Classification:
                                        Schedule:

Brand names: Dosage forms:

Indications and usage:

                                        Dosage:

Generic name: Classification:
                                        Schedule:

Brand names: Dosage forms:

Indications and usage:

                                        Dosage:

Generic name: Classification:
                                        Schedule:

Brand names: Dosage forms:

Indications and usage:

                                        Dosage:

Adverse reactions/side effects:

Contraindications:

Adverse reactions/side effects:

Contraindications:

Adverse reactions/side effects:

Contraindications:

Adverse reactions/side effects:

Contraindications:

Generic name:

Classification:
Schedule:

Brand names:

Dosage forms:

Indications and usage:

Dosage:

Generic name:

Classification:
Schedule:

Brand names:

Dosage forms:

Indications and usage:

Dosage:

Generic name:

Classification:
Schedule:

Brand names:

Dosage forms:

Indications and usage:

Dosage:

Generic name:

Classification:
Schedule:

Brand names:

Dosage forms:

Indications and usage:

Dosage:

Adverse reactions/side effects:

Contraindications:

Adverse reactions/side effects:

Contraindications:

Adverse reactions/side effects:

Contraindications:

Adverse reactions/side effects:

Contraindications:

Generic name:

Classification:
Schedule:

Brand names:

Dosage forms:

Indications and usage:

Dosage:

Generic name:

Classification:
Schedule:

Brand names:

Dosage forms:

Indications and usage:

Dosage:

Brand names:

Dosage forms:

Generic name:

Classification:
Schedule:

Indications and usage:

Dosage:

Brand names:

Dosage forms:

Generic name:

Classification:
Schedule:

Indications and usage:

Dosage:

Adverse reactions/side effects:

Contraindications:

Adverse reactions/side effects:

Contraindications:

Contraindications:

Adverse reactions/side effects:

Contraindications:

Adverse reactions/side effects:

Contraindications:

Generic name:

Classification:
Schedule:

Brand names:

Dosage forms:

Indications and usage:

Dosage:

Generic name:

Classification:
Schedule:

Brand names:

Dosage forms:

Indications and usage:

Dosage:

Generic name:

Classification:
Schedule:

Brand names:

Dosage forms:

Indications and usage:

Dosage:

Generic name:

Classification:
Schedule:

Brand names:

Dosage forms:

Indications and usage:

Dosage:

Adverse reactions/side effects:

Contraindications:

Adverse reactions/side effects:

Contraindications:

Adverse reactions/side effects:

Contraindications:

Adverse reactions/side effects:

Contraindications:

Generic name:

Classification:
Schedule:

Brand names:

Dosage forms:

Indications and usage:

Dosage:

Generic name:

Classification:
Schedule:

Brand names:

Dosage forms:

Indications and usage:

Dosage:

Generic name:

Classification:
Schedule:

Brand names:

Dosage forms:

Indications and usage:

Dosage:

Generic name:

Classification:
Schedule:

Brand names:

Dosage forms:

Indications and usage:

Dosage: